The

D1561989

Scientific Basis
for
Selected
Environmental
Medicine
Techniques

by

Sherry A. Rogers, M.D.

Novabiomedical
Novabio.com

Dear Informed Healthcare Consumer:

The following explanations and references have been helpful for insurance companies, attorneys, physicians, patients, small claims courts, and institutions in understanding that there is a wealth of scientific backup for environmental medicine. It has also been useful for Medicare and Medicaid to explain the departure from drug-oriented medicine into this biochemically and cause-oriented approach to medicine.

Current medical practice is fast becoming a computerized cookbook, with dictation of what drugs and surgery should be used and the prescribing of medications by rote. In contrast, environmental medicine requires thinking, biochemical knowledge, detective work, and finding the cause of symptoms so that they can be healed once and for all. For a headache is not an aspirin deficiency.

Most drugs in the PDR say "mechanism of action unknown," but indeed the mechanism is known or they could not have passed the FDA as safe for human use. It turns out that every place a drug works, there is usually an environmental trigger and a biochemical defect, and one of the aims of environmental medicine is to identify these environmental triggers and biochemical defects and correct them. This is a logical substitute for a lifetime of medication that ignores the biochemical defect so that it inevitably goes on to cause further symptoms.

Lastly, environmental medicine necessitates education of the patient as well as his responsible participation in his health. It has long been recognized that such things as responsible diet selections and life style choices have a great bearing on health. For after all, health is not a birth right. It is a right way of living.

1

THE SCIENTIFIC BASIS FOR SELECTED ENVIRONMENTAL MEDICINE TECHNIQUES

TABLE OF CONTENTS

HISTORY AND PHYSICAL
Reference:

Agency for Toxic Substances and Disease Registry,Department of Health and Human Services, Public Health Service, Atlanta, GA. Obtaining an exposure history. AMER FAMILY PHYSICIAN Sept. 1, 1993;48:3,483-491.

"Abstract: Because many **environmental diseases manifest as common medical problems or have nonspecific symptoms,** an exposure history is vital for correct diagnosis. The primary care physician can—by obtaining a thorough exposure history—play an important role in detecting, treating, and preventing diseases caused by toxic exposure. The exposure history consists of three parts: exposure survey, which includes information about current and past exposure and health and safety practices at work; work history, including all past jobs and military service; and environmental history, which includes information about the home environment."

"Few physicians routinely elicit information about the patient's home, workplace, or community environment as part of the demographic and social history. In a study of primary care practice in an academic setting, only 24% of 625 charts included any mention of the patient's occupation. Only 2% of the charts included information about toxic exposures, duration of present employment, and former occupation. Most physicians have had little training or practice in obtaining a work and exposure history."

This government agency states that to give drugs without an environmental investigation results in inappropriate treatment. Again we quote from the government paper:

"Most environmental and occupational diseases either manifest as common medical problems or have nonspecific symptoms. It is the etiology that distinguishes a disorder as an environmental illness. **Unless an exposure history is pursued by the physician, the etiologic diagnosis may be missed, treatment may be inappropriate, and exposure may continue.**"

"This article describes the investigation of environmental and occupational illness. The aim is not to demonstrate all exposure possibilities but to show the principles and process of investigating the disease etiology."

"**An exposure history should be obtained for every patient. It is of particular importance if the patient's illness occurs at an atypical age or is unresponsive to treatment.** The physician must also keep in mind that many organ systems are affected by toxic exposure. The latency period from exposure to manifestation of symptoms can vary, ranging from immediate to delayed (hours or days) to prolonged (decades)."

Therefore, according to the U.S. Government Department of Health and Human Services agency, it is really almost malpractice not to do an environmental workup on a patient, regardless of symptoms. Furthermore it is customary for most physicians to be deficient in this area, which has grave consequences. It makes the difference between whether or not the cause of symptoms is found or a lifetime of costly, potentially dangerous, and unnecessary medications are prescribed.

In fact, one reference refers to the fact that to ignore taking such a history may constitute malpractice: "Legal precedent is currently incomplete. However, the liability of the physician should be cause for concern if a correctable

6

occupational hazard is ignored or if a potentially compensable disability is inadequately evaluated".

The Occupational and Environmental Health Committee of the American Lung Association of San Diego and Imperial Countries, Taking the occupational history. ANN INT MED 1983; 99: 641-651.

LABORATORY

It is clear that biochemical defects accompany illness/disease/symptoms. For example low thyroid function tests accompany hypothyroidism. Elevated liver function tests accompany hepatitis. Likewise, such symptoms as chronic fatigue, chemical sensitivity, toxic encephalopathy, or really any malfunction must be accompanied by biochemical defects.

Nutritional Deficiencies Are Common

It is a known biochemical fact that for every place a drug works, there are nutrient replacements that can correct the deficiencies so that the symptoms are modified, often to the point of disappearing and the drug is no longer needed. To complicate matters, in this era there are numerous reasons for the increase in nutrient deficiencies among the population.

(1) Because we are the first generation to ever eat so many processed foods, we are low in nutrients. Scores of papers (many of them government surveys) demonstrate that at least half of the average population is low in such necessary nutrients as magnesium, chromium, copper, and much more. For example, U.S. government surveys(SCIENCE NEWS, 1988) show the average American diet only provides 40%, or less than half, of the magnesium a person needs in a day. This deficiency alone can cause or contribute to over forty different symptoms from headache, chronic fatigue, insomnia, anxiety, asthma, and cardiac arrhythmia to chronic back pain or sudden cardiac death (INTERN MED WORLD REP, 1990).

Schroeder's studies (1969) have shown that when we go from whole grains down to bleached flour products, we lose approximately 80% of the nutrients. Indeed, the work of processing foods has significantly lowered the nutrient base for a major part of the population. When these deficiencies reach a critical level, then we have symptoms.

Furthermore, people's food selections, which often include fewer whole grains and vegetables and more processed foods, drive the nutrient basis even lower. If that were not enough, (2) we are also the first generation of man ever exposed to so many chemicals. The average person has to detoxify over 500 chemicals in his everyday home and office environment. The work of detoxifying these chemicals that outgas from furniture, carpet, clothes, toiletries, business supplies, paper products, machines, construction materials, industrial and auto exhaust plus much more actually uses up nutrients (Parke 1982).

For example, every time we walk through a grocery store or an office building and detoxify one molecule of pesticide, we use up or throw away forever certain detox nutrients. For example, every molecule of pesticide detoxified throws away one molecule of glutathione and magnesium. Therefore, there are 2 major reasons why this generation is at greater risk and probability of having nutrient deficiencies. And a mountain of scientific studies bears this out.

Anonymous, Magnesium deficiency; a new risk factor for sudden cardiac death. INTERN MED WORLD REP, 5:9, 18, 1990

Schroeder Ja, Nason AP, Tipton IH; Essential Metals in Man, Magnesium, J CHRON DIS 21: 815-841, 1969

Parke DV, Mechanisms of Chemical Toxicity, REGULATORY TOXICOLOGY AND PHARMACOLOGY, 2, 267-286, 1982

Anonymous,New Misgivings About Magnesium,SCIENCE NEWS 133: 32, 356, 1988

Nutritional Medicine Saves Money
reference:

Delmi M., Rapin CH, Bengoa JM, Delmas PD, Vasey IT, et al, Dietary supplementation in elderly patients with fractured neck of the femur. LANCET, 335; 1013-1016, 1990

In this study 59 patients, all with a hip fracture and median age of 82, were divided into 2 groups. One had a multiple vitamin-mineral given and the other did not. The group with the nutrients had an average hospital stay of 22 days. The group without the supplement had an average hospital stay of 44 days. Double the time and more than double the expense. Plus the supplemented group had half the deaths, half the complications, and half as much medication. There is no contest, and enormous savings of money and lives. Yet this is still not routine.

Correction of Nutrient Deficiencies Treats Symptoms

Furthermore, there are literally thousands of references in the scientific literature detailing how the identification and correction of nutrient deficiencies have eliminated symptoms for which otherwise, medications would have been prescribed for years or for a lifetime. The unfortunate part in the use of medications is that they cost money, have a laundry list of side effects, use up further nutrients in the work of the body detoxifying them, and they rarely terminate the illness, but merely mask or cover up symptoms. They allow the underlying cause, such as a magnesium deficiency, to go undetected so that it can escalate and go on to cause other symptoms, such as sudden cardiac arrest from magnesium deficiency.

10

Furthermore, medication uses up detox nutrients, for every medication is also a foreign chemical and has to be metabolized or detoxified. So it drives the system even lower and depletes people further, setting them up for new illnesses, worsening of the existing illnesses, and making them prime targets for eventual fatal cardiovascular diseases or cancer.

As an example of how one nutrient can cause multiple symptoms, lets look at magnesium:

Magnesium As An Example Of The Diverse Symptoms One Mineral Deficiency Can Cause

Let's look at one out of over 40 essential nutrients to see how prevalent deficiencies are, and how under diagnosed, and how crucial to disease and to disease progression they are.

The JOURNAL OF AMERICAN MEDICAL ASSOCIATION(Whang R, 1990) shows that 90% of physicians do not even think of ordering a magnesium test, even when over 54% of 1033 hospitalized patients are low and many die from it.

Other studies show that magnesium deficiency can cause bronchial spasm and result in asthma. It can cause abnormal ability to metabolize cholesterol and therefore cause hypercholesterolemia. It can lead to spasm in the gut and irritable bowel syndrome. It can cause fatigue. It can cause or exacerbate chemical sensitivity, cystitis, chronic back problems, hypertension, cardiac arrthythmia, PMS, and much more.

You can go either way. You can search magnesium and find hundreds of articles on various conditions that are improved once magnesium deficiency is discovered and corrected. Likewise, you can search one disease and find

11

multiple nutrient deficiencies whose diagnoses and corrections have led to the termination of the symptoms. We will give an example of each.

For example, papers in the literature show that often asthmatics are low in magnesium, B12, or omega 3 essential fatty acids. Likewise, high cholesterol can be caused by the inability to properly metabolize cholesterol, such as occurs with deficiencies of chromium, manganese, magnesium, copper, and much more. And obviously, such broad multi-system and multi- metabolic problems such as chronic fatigue and chemical sensitivity can have a host of deficiencies. The diagnosis of fatigue alone warrants looking for every nutrient there is, because fatigue is one of the most common symptoms for a deficiency of any nutrient.

Likewise, chemical sensitivity merely reflects the inability of a person to metabolize everyday chemicals as efficiently as the rest of the world. These people have difficulty doing so because they are deficient in the nutrients that run the detox pathways. Bare minimum should be an rbc manganese, rbc zinc, rbc copper (all in super oxide dismutase) and a magnesium loading test. Also important would be an rbc potassium and rbc calcium. When these sensitive indicators are abnormally low, it suggests that the potassium and/or calcium pumps have been damaged, such as by years of trans fatty acids, everyday chemicals, or even antihistamines. Since these pumps lie in this lipid bilayer or sandwich, it is indicative of further damage in the cell membrane (which is like the computer keyboard of the cell) which dictates many disease states and symptoms including allergies, auto- immune phenomena, arteriosclerosis, cancer, and more.

MYTH: If you eat a balanced diet, you cannot get deficient

A common myth perpetrated only by those ignorant of current biochemical literature is that "If you eat a balanced diet, you can't get deficient." This commonly offered medical advice overlooks the fact that the majority of the SAD (standard American diet) is processed, leaving 25-75% of the original nutrients in food. Recall, U.S. Government surveys show, for example that the average American only gets 40% or less than half the magnesium he needs in a day. And here is an example of one mineral responsibile for a significant amount of hypertension, cardiac arrhythmia, fatigue and even sudden death.

We are the first generation to ever be continually detoxifying such an unprecedented number of daily chemicals (over 500 average). Add to that the fact that the work of detoxification loses or uses up nutrients, and it is really a tribute to the design of our bodies that we do as well as we do. In a Food and Drug Administration study to analyze 234 foods over 2 years, they found the average American diet to have less than 80% of the RDA (recommended daily allowance) of one or more: calcium, magnesium, iron, zinc, copper, and manganese (Pennington, 1986).

In one study of patients admitted to an acute medical service, 23-50% had undiscovered deficiencies, and this was not a sophisticated analysis (Roubenoff, 1987). When other studies have demonstrated magnesium deficiency in well over 50% of the population (Rogers, 1991, Whang, 1990, Rea, 1986,) it behooves all physicians to not condemn any symptom to a lifetime of medications without ruling out deficiencies. For as you can appreciate, even the most seemingly minor of symptoms, like anxiety, insomnia, or depression can herald a magnesium or other nutrient deficit that can begin to insidiously disrupt arterial and cardiac integrity and consequently increase the vulnerability to life-threatening events (Seelig, 1989).

But if a magnesium deficiency of anxiety, for example , is unknowingly masked with a seemingly harmless tranquilizer, the opportunity to prevent more serious sequelae is lost or at best delayed. Magnesium deficiency can also lead to sudden death and reduce the chances of successful resuscitation.

BEHIND EVERY SYMPTOM IS A BIOCHEMICAL ABNORMALITY --- OFTEN A DIAGNOSABLE AND TREATABLE DEFICIENCY

Every symptom, regardless of how difficult to treat by "drug-oriented medicine, must have a biochemical defect. Otherwise, how could a chemical drug suppress the symptom?

Vasculitis is an example of a symptom complex that is difficult to diagnose and nearly impossible to treat. There is generally no known cause and there certainly are few effective treatments, as the prognosis is bleak.

Yet in the heart of the citrus belt of the US, researchers from Tampa reported on several cases of serious vasculitis that were due to vitamin C deficiency. And these patients, before the correct diagnosis was made, were subjected to life-threatening doses of steroids and therapeutic agents in attempt to just control the vasculitis.

Alderman Hm, Wallach PM, Gutienez F, Kreitze SM, Seleznick MJ, Espinoza C6, Espinoza LR: Scurvy resembling cutaneous vasculitis, CUTIS 54:111-114, Aug 1994. You can begin to appreciate how many malpractice cases would stem from drug-oriented medicine that fails to look for treatable biochemical causes, and for cases against insurance companies that condone chemotherapeutic agents like cyclophosphamide for treatment of vasculitis, but will not cover lab tests to check nutrient biochemistry. These chemotherapy-type drugs can cause cancer, or can cause death as a side effect, long before the drug has a chance to induce a cancer.

Make no mistake about it. We are in a dangerous era where the correctable biochemistry that underlies disease is being ignored. Meanwhile, drugs are used which ignore the cause and actually help the sick get sicker, quicker, and at great expense.

For example, files bulge with scientific papers showing how biochemical defects must underly every medical problem. For example, high cholesterol in many cases is merely the result of nutrient deficiencies in the cholesterol metabolism pathway: magnesium, chromium, vitamin C, and copper deficiencies are all examples that can cause it.

But the U.S. government FDA studied 234 foods that make up the majority of the American diet and found that it provided only 80% of the recommended daily allowances (RDA) of copper, for example.

And so it should come as no surprise that a U.S. government National Institute of Health study showed that 81% of people had less than two thirds RDA for copper each day.

No wonder a study of 270 U.S. Navy SEAL trainees (supposedly very fit young men) showed that 37% of them were deficient in copper. And no wonder then that arteriosclerotic lesions are found in U.S. teenage soldiers at autopsy and that arteriosclerosis is the number one cause of death and

15

disease in the U.S.. And yet we still treat high cholesterol with cholesterol metabolism blockers. And we treat hypertension with antihypertensives that increase the loss of these minerals and further raise lipids! Yes you understood correctly. The very medicines that are commonly prescribed for control of hypertension actually cause high cholesterol. Again because the cause is being ignored and the symptom hidden or suppressed by a drug:

Lardinois CK, Neuman SL, The effects of antihypertensive agents on serum lipids and lipoproteins. ARCH INTERN MED 148:1280-1288, 1988

In Summary:

* Deficiencies are so common, they are the rule, not the exception.

* The average diet and daily chemical exposures are the main cause.

* Deficiencies of nutrients are behind most symptoms that are customarily masked with medications.

* When drugs are used, the opportunity to find the cause is lost.

* A lifetime of drugs is unnecessarily prescribed

* Most importantly, the ignored cause of the symptoms has to cause further symptoms or disease, and more quickly.

* There is no logical, scientific, ethical or financial reason for an insurance company to deny payment

for tests to detect biochemical abnormalities that underly symptoms.

Cannon LA, Heiselman DE, Dougherty JM, Jones J. Magnesium levels in cardiac arrest victims: Relationship between magnesium levels and successful resuscitation. ANN EMERG MED 16, 1195-1198, 1987

Cox IM, Campbell MJ, Dowson D, Red blood cell magnesium and chronic fatigue syndrome. LANCET 337, 757-760, 1991

Delmi M, Rapin CH, Bengoa JM, Delmas PD, Vasey H, et al., Dietary supplementation in elderly patients with fractured neck of the femur. LANCET 335: 1013-1016, 1990

Iseri LT, French JH, Magnesium: Nature's physiologic calcium blocker. AM HEART J 108:1, 188-192, 1984

Leary WP, Reyes AJ, Magnesium and sudden death, SA MED J 64, 697-698, 1983

Marier JR, Magnesium content of the food supply in the modern-day world. MAGNESIUM 5:1-8, 1986

Marino PL, The hidden threat of magnesium deficiency, INTERN MED 12:6, 32-46, 1991

Nicar MJ, Pak CYC, Oral magnesium deficiency, causes and effects. HOSPITAL PRACTICE 116A-116P, 1987

Pennington JA, Young BE, The selected minerals in foods surveyed from 1982 to 1984, J AMER DIETETIC ASSOC 86:7, 876, July 1986

Purvis Jr, Cummings DM, Effect of oral magnesium supplementations on selected cardiovascular risk factors in non-insulin-dependent diabetics. ARCH FAM MED. 3: 503-508, 1994

Rea WJ, Johnson AR, Smiley RE, Maynard B, Dawkins-Brown): Magnesium deficiency in patients with chemical sensitivity, CLIN ECOL, 4:1, 17-20, 1986

Rhinehart RA, Magnesium metabolism: A review with special reference to the relationship between intracellular content and serum levels ARCH INT MED 148, 2415-2420, 1988

Rogers SA, Unrecognized Magnesium Deficiency Masquerades as Diverse Symptoms. Evaluation of an Oral Magnesium Challenge Test. INTERNAT CLIN NUTR REV 11:3, 117-125, 1991

Roubenoff R, et al, Malnutrition among hospitalized patients: Problem of physician awareness, ARCH INTERN MED 147:1462- 1465, 1987

Siscovick DS, Raghunathan TE, et al, Diuretic therapy for hypertension and the risk of primary cardiac arrest. N ENGL J MED 1994; 330: 1852-7

Seelig M, Cardiovascular consequences of magnesium deficiency and loss: Pathogenesis, prevalence, and manifestations-magnesium and chloride loss in refractory potassium repletion. AM J CARDIOL 53,4g-21g, 1989

Seelig CB, Magnesium deficiency in hypertension uncovered by magnesium load retention. J AM CLIN NUTR 8:5,455, abs. 113, 1989

Singh RB, Cameron EA, Relation of myocardial magnesium

deficiency to sudden death in ischaemic heart disease. AM HEART J 103:3, 399-450, 1982

Warram JH, Lori LMB, Valsania P, Christlieb AR, Krolewski AS, Excess mortality associated with diuretic therapy in diabetes mellitus, ARCH INTERN MED 151, 1350-1356, 1991

Whang R, Ryder KW, Frequency of hypomagnesemia and hypermagnesemia, requested versus routine, JAMA 2634, 3063- 3064, 1990

So it is readily apparent that vastly improved health, productivity, and reduced cost can result from a biochemical approach to symptoms. And this extends to nearly all problems, even cancers.

For example, when everything has been done for certain types of bladder cancers, within 2 years 80% of the people have a recurrence of their cancer. However, those who were given 4 simple vitamins, the recurrence rate dropped from 80% to 40% or in half!

reference:
Lamm DL, Riggs DR, Shriver JS, Van Gilder PF, Rach JF, DeHaven JI, Mega -dose vitamins in bladder cancer; A double-blind clinical trial, J UROL, 21-76, Jan 1994

When a non-sophisticated prescription of only 4 vitamins cuts the recurrence rate of cancer in half, this is pretty dramatic evidence of what types of savings and health improvements are documented for other diseases.

Nutrient Deficiencies Are Part of the Cause
of Chemical Sensitivity

Likewise, victims of chemical sensitivity have impaired xenobiotic (foreign chemical) detoxication (metabolism or processing). And correcting this can allow them to recover. There are literally volumes of books detailing this medical chemistry. A small example follows. Just bear in mind that these books cite hundreds of scientific references, as well as describing the mechanisms.

Jakoby WB, ENZYMATIC BASIS OF DETOXICATION Vol I, Acadamic Press, 24/28 Oval Road, London NW17DX, 1980:

This book goes through the major detoxication enzymes of phase 1 and phase 2, including alcohol dehydrogenases, aldehyde oxidase, cytochrome P-450, superoxide dismutases, glutathione peroxidase and monoamine oxidases.

Vol II, Ibid, 1980:

This volume details the congugation pathways.

Hathcock JN, Editor (and affiliated with the FDA in Washington DC), MICRO NUTRIENTS IN DETOXICATION (p14-39 in NUTRITIONAL TOXICOLOGY, Academic Press, Orlando, 1987):

This book also details how vitamins E and A contribute to the stability of membranes, which, of course, includes endoplasmic reticular membranes where the work of chemical (xenobiotic) detoxification occurs. As well, it explains that vitamin C is a major detoxification agent protecting against hydrocarbons, pesticides, heavy metals, demoting

20

carcinogenicity and correcting toxicity and improving drug metabolism.

For example, vitamin B2 supplies the reducing equivalent to cytochrome P-450 (NADPH). Vitamin B1 is important in carbohydrate metabolism, for example, in people with chronic fatigue as well as those with mental symptoms, heavy metal disease, and pesticide toxicity. B6 is important in revving up drug detoxification to decrease toxicity. B12 is likewise important in the detoxification of cyanide, which is a common component of everyday pesticides, not to mention carbon tetrachloride and other chemicals that can be included as part of the inert ingredients of pesticides and also are common solvents in the industrial work place.

Caldwell J, Jacoby WB, Eds; Impact of Nutrition on Detoxication in BIOLOGICAL BASIS OF DETOXICATION, Academic Press, New York, 1983, Pg 297-306:

In here, the inter- relatedness of nutrients is brought out. For example, vitamin A protects vitamin E; vitamin C is important for regeneration of minerals into the active or reduced form and does the same with vitamin E, reducing it to the active tocopherol form again. Lipid peroxidation can lead to decreased oxidase activity and without antioxidants to protect these membranes, further detox pathways are compromised and the individual is on a downward roll or starts to exhibit what is called the spreading phenomenon where he gets progressively sicker. He gets more and more symptoms, consults a stable of specialists, but never gets well until he consults someone who identifies the biochemical defects.

Feuer G, de la Iglesia FA, MOLECULAR BIOCHEMISTRY OF HUMAN DISEASE, Vol I, CRC Press, Boca Raton, Florida, 1985 Pg 77- 79.

This work demonstrates again the continual loss of nutrients in the work of detoxification, such as the loss of glutathione and phosphatidyl ethanolamine, as examples. Again, remember that the work of living in this polluted century uses up nutrients daily in everyone.

Bland J, Brally A. Nutritional Upregulation of Hepatic Detoxification Enzymes. J App NUTR 1992: 44 (3.4) 2-15

There Is Justification To Look For Nutrient Deficiencies For Every Symptom And In Every Disease

In order to keep this monograph small, we will have had to omit thousands of references. To summarize the main points that these papers support:

1. Nutrient deficiencies are the rule, not the exception.

2. Every symptom or disease has to have biochemical (nutrient) deficiencies associated with it.

3. Taking medication further depletes nutrients.

4. Nutrient deficiencies cause symptoms and classi fiable disease that are treated with drugs.

5. Correction of these deficiencies can turn off symptoms if the deficiency alone is a major cause. Otherwise the other contributing factors must be dealt with.

6. One nutrient deficiency alone can cause over forty different symptoms. Each nutrient is re sponsible for specific enzymes and pathways.

7. Due to individual biochemistry, the same symptoms are not caused by the same deficiencies and like wise the same deficiencies do not cause the same symptoms in everyone.

8. In view of the medical literature to date, it is nearly malpractice to fail to investigate the biochemistry before resorting to chronic drugs. For these drugs, aside from their side effects, potentiate the underlying cause of symptoms and foster the development of new symptoms. Furthermore, drugs use up precious (detox) nutrients, adding to one's deficiencies.

Vitamin Deficiencies Also Can Cause Conditions Treated By Surgery

Sometimes people unknowledgable about nutritional bio-chemistry can understand how deficiencies might cause a symptom like fatigue, but cannot see how they could relate to other conditions, such as surgical conditions, for example. So let's look at a simple example:

For over a decade it has been known that a pyridoxine, or vitamin B6 deficiency can be the sole cause for carpal tunnel syndrome in some people. And by correcting this, no surgery on the wrist is needed. And when the B6 deficiency is corrected, it does not silently continue to contribute to depression, arteriosclerosis, hyperemesis gravidarum (nausea of pregnancy), PMS, allergy, and other conditions that have also been caused by B6 deficiency.

Folkers K, Ellis JM, Watanbe T, Saji S, Kaji M: Biochemical evidence for a deficiency of vitamin B6 in the carpal tunnel syndrome based on a cross-over clinical study. PROC NATL ACAD SCI USA 75:3410-3412, 1978.

Ellis JM, Folkers K, Levy M, Shizukuishi S, Lewandowski J, Nishii S, Schubert H, Ulrich R: Response of vitamin B6 deficiency and the carpal tunnel syndrome to pyridoxine. PROC NATL ACAD SCI USA 79:7494-7498, 1982.

Ellis JM: Treatment of carpal tunnel syndrome with vitamin B6. SOUTH MED J 80:882-884, 1987.

Ellis JM, Folkers K: Clinical aspects of treatment of carpal tunnel syndrome with vitamin B6, in VITAMIN B6, Dakshinamurti K (ed), ANN NEW YORK ACAD SCI 585:302-320, 1990.

Minerals, Vitamins, Amino Acids, And Essential Fatty Acids All Run The Body Chemistry

So we have given examples of how deficient the diet is, and how deficient the population is, how deficiencies can cause nearly any symptom and how they underlie nearly all disease and symptoms.

We looked at magnesium as an example of a **mineral**, because it is in over 300 enzymes and pathways. And government studies show that the average person does not even get half of the amount he needs in a day. As well, similar circumstances exist for other nutrients, for example, government studies show the average American gets less than 1mg of copper a day, and the requirement is 2-4mg a day. Copper is in 21 enzymes, and its deficiency can lead to aneurysms, depression, hypoglycemia, fatigue, chemical sensitivity, high cholesterol, arthralgia, and much more. We could go on and explore each nutrient in similar fashion.

24

Cox IM, Campbell MJ, Dowson D, Red Blood Cell Magnesium and Chronic Fatgue Syndrome, LANCET 1991; 337. 757-760
Klevay LM, Reck SJ, Barcome DP: Evidence of dietary copper and zinc deficiencies. JAMA 241:1916-1918, 1979.

National Research Council: "Recommended Dietary Allowances", Washington, DC, Nat Acad Sci, 1980.

Holden JM, Wolf WR, Mertz W: Zinc and copper in self selected diets. J AM DIET ASSOC 75:23-28, 1979.

Likewise zinc is in over 90 enzymes, and has a broad range of effects from digestive and metabolic enzymes to protection against infection, cancer and chemical sensitivity.

Zinc: A public health problem. NUTR & M.D., 1992; 18:4

Rogers SA: Zinc deficiency as a model for developing chemical sensitivity. INTERN CLIN NUTR REV, 10:1, 253, Jan 1990.

And we looked at vitamin B6 as an example of a **vitamin**, but much more has been written about vitamin C, which has anti- histaminic properties, is anti-inflammatory, accelerates drug metabolism, recycles vitamins and minerals that have been used up in body reactions so that they are useful again, etc. Single textbooks fully referenced cannot cover all of its chemistry. We could go on for all the vitamins.

Johnston CS, Martin LJ, Cai X, Antihistamine effect of supplemental ascorbic acid and neutrophil chemotaxis. J AMER CLIN NUTR 1992; 11:172-176.

Likewise, **amino acids** are important. Taurine has corrected cardiac failure, cardiac arrhythmias, seizure disorders, it cysteine (its metabolic source in the body) is used up and thrown away with the work of detoxification, which every person's body is doing every moment of their lives.

Barbeau A, Huxtable RJ, TAURINE AND NEUROLOGICAL DISORDERS, Raven Press NY, 1978

Richardson MA, Ed, AMINO ACIDS IN PSYCHIATRIC DISEASE, American Psychiatric Press, Wash, DC, 1984: This book points up the variation in amino acids from person to person and how they can be diagnosed and corrected. This variability is known, because that is why there are many different types of antidepressants and tranquilizers. Everyone does not have the same biochemical defect.

Likewise, many diseases thought of as hopeless or due to lack of moral fiber, like alcoholism as an example, can be corrected by identifying the biochemical defects.

Blum K, Trachtenberg MC, Neurogenic deficits caused by alcoholism: Restoration by SAAVE, a neuronutrient intervention adjunct, J PSYCHOACTIVE DRUGS, 20:3, Jul-Sept 1988, 297-313.

Larson JM, ALCOHOLISM - THE BIOCHEMICAl CONNECTION, Villard Books, NY, 1992.

Essential fatty acids not only control the inflammatory response (every disease that ends in "-itis" involves inflammation), but the whole response of the body in terms of whether it develops allergies, arthritis, auto-immune diseases, chemical sensitivity, cancer, or arteriosclerosis. NEW ENGLAND JOURNAL OF MEDICINE studies (Aug 16, 1990) show that eating of hydrogentated oils (the main oils in processed foods like fried foods, breads, eggs substitutes, mayonnaise, salad dressings, margarines) actually displaces the preferred essential fatty acids (eicosapentaenoic, for example) and accelerates the changes that cause arthritis, arteriosclerosis, and other diseases including cancers---- the main causes of disease and death in the U.S..

Magnesium Loading Test
As An Example of One Type of Specialized Test

A study of the medical literature reveals that serum and RBC magnesium tests miss identifying some people with magnesium deficiency. Therefore, a before and after urine assay after oral or parenteral loading is the preferred test.

Since the **Journal of the American Medical Association** shows that over 54% of patients hospitalized were low in magnesium and U.S. Government surveys (SCIENCE NEWS 1988) showed that the average American diet provides 40% or less than half of the amount of magnesium that a person needs in a day, magnesium deficiency is very important. Couple this with the fact that magnesium is necessary in over 300 enzyme reactions and can cause over forty symptoms including sudden cardiac death, and it becomes child's play to understand why magnesium should be checked for in any patient who has any symptoms whatsoever. And multiple publications make these same recommendations. For it is close to malpractice to overlook a magnesium deficiency before sentencing a patient to a lifetime of medication that allows the physician to merely mask or cover up the symptoms and the deficiency, and thereby hasten the possibility of sudden cardiac death.

In Summary:

*   Magnesium as an example of one of over 40 essential nutrients, is deficient in over half the populus in many studies.

* It can cause over 40 symptoms

* Calcium channel blockers, tranquilizers, antidepres sants, bronchodilators, anti-arrhythmia drugs, muscle relaxants, intestinal anti-spasmodics, and anti- hypertensives are just a sample of the drugs used to cover up magnesium deficiency symptoms.

* To continue to use drugs to "control" a symptom can hasten the onset of worse and new symptoms and even sudden cardiac death.

* The serum magnesium is an inferior test as it misses many deficiencies.

* The magnesium loading test is superior.

Baker SM, Magnesium in Primary Case and Preventive medicine: clinical correlation of magnesium loading studies. MAGNES & TRACE ELEMENTS, 1991-92: 10: 251-262

Fortunately most minerals are much less cumbersome to assess, the best assay being intracellular. This is because of homeostasis and the fact that there is also a greater concentration intracellularly than in the serum or plasma assays. The red blood cell (rbc) is the most sensitive and accurate intracellular assay for most minerals that is the most accessable. No tissue biopsies are needed, merely a venipuncture blood sample. But white cells can be used as well.

Patrick J, Dervish C: Leucocyte zinc in the assessment of zinc status, CRC CR17 REV CLIN LAB SCI, 20: 95-104. 1984

Jones RB, Keeling PWN, Hilton PJ, et al. The relationship between leukocyte and muscle zinc in health and disease, CLIN. SCI, 60: 237-239, 1981

If the slightest doubt should remain about the medical correctness and necessity of evaluating and correcting the nutritional status of the patient, see the Legal section on non- prescription drugs.

ENVIRONMENTAL CONTROLS

Creating the Allergy-Free Oasis

Classic in the control of allergy has always been avoidance. More and more information is in the literature describing the importance of doing environmental controls so that the environment is not as noxious. Foremost is exposure of mold plates or petri dishes to find out how much mold is around, since mold allergy can mimic chemical sensitivity as well as any other disease. When we know that someone is sensitive to dust, mites and mold, it makes sense to remove carpets, since the nap on a carpet can hold as much as 100 times the square surface area of dust, mite and mold as can a flat wooden floor.

Likewise, air depollution devices or air cleaners, whether they be hepa, electrostatic, or other mechanisms, remove significant amounts of dust, mites and mold from the environment. Chemically sensitive patients are sensitive to formaldehyde sizing and color fastness of bed linens as well as the outgassing of formaldehyde, pesticides, and fire retardants from mattresses. Cotton bedding and mattress pads, and sometimes even cotton for the mattress themselves is important as well as for pillows. The goal is to make the bedroom in which the person spends 1/3 of his life an environmental oasis; a place to which he can escape and, so to speak, regroup or improve and heal in order to be ready for the onslaught of chemicals from the 21st century world the next day.

Furthermore, more studies show that many environmental pollutants come from the ambient outside air and so it must be filtered before it enters the house.

Neher JO, Coenig JQ. Health effects of outdoor air pollu-

Wickman M, Gravesen S, Nordvall SL, Pershagen G, Sundell J.Indoor viable dust-bound microfungi in relation to residential characteristics, living habits, and symptoms in atopic and controlled children. J ALLERGY & CLIN IMMUNOL. 1992;89:752-9.

Sanda T, Yasue T, Oohashi M, Yasue A. Effectiveness of house dust mite allergen avoidance through clean room therapy in patients with atopic dermatitis. JACI 1992;89:653-7.

Bardana EJ, Air pollution in the home: What to advise your patients, J Resp Dis 15:7, 612-618, 1984.

Books are recommended which teach a great deal about various aspects of environmental controls:

Randolf T, Moss RW, AN ALTERNATIVE APPROACH TO ALLERGIES, Bantam Books, NY 1982

Rousseau D, Rea WJ, Enwright J, YOUR HOME AND YOUR HEALTH AND WELL-BEING Hartley & Marks, 3663 W. Broadway, Vancouver BC, V6R2B8, 1988

Rogers SA, THE E.I. SYNDROME, Prestige Publ., Syracuse, NY 1986

Rogers SA, TIRED OR TOXIC?, Prestige Publ., Syracuse NY, 1990

Rapp DJ, IS THIS YOUR CHILD?, WM Morrow & Co., NY 1991

Golas N, golbitz FG, COPING WITH YOUR ALLERGIES,

Simon & Schuster NY, 1986

Dadd DL, NON-TOXIC AND NATURAL, Jeremy Torcher, Los Angeles, 1986

Furthermore, many other adjuncts are of proven benefit. There is a world-wide increased incidence of near-fatal asthma attacks, but studies remind us that the instruction in the use of an inexpensive peak-flow meter can help deter these.

K, Kuchi Y, Obabe S, Tamura G, et al: Chemosensitivity and perception of dyspnea in patients with a history of near-fatal asthma. N ENGL J MED 330: 1329-1334, May 12 1994

And on the flip side, there are items sold that the patient should be advised against wasting money on

Huss RW, Huss K Squire EN, et al, Mite allergen control with acaricide fails. J ALLERGY CLIN IMMUNOL 1994; 94: 27-32

The United States government's EPA recommends extensive environmental controls be taught to patients regarding storage of home chemicals, water filters on kitchen and bathroom taps, discontinuing room air freshners and smoking, installing air cleaners, airing of dry-cleaned clothes, etc:

EPA, Project Summary, The Total Exposure Assessment Methodology (TEAM) Study, Wallace LA, Office of Acid Deposition, Environmental Monitoring and Quality Assurance, Wash DC, 20460, EPA /600/s6-87/002, pp 1-14, Sept 1987

MOLD PLATES OR PETRI DISHES

The first principle of any allergic treatment is avoidance and you cannot avoid or clean up what you are not aware of. It is common knowledge in the mycologic field (the study of molds) that among the thousands of species of fungi (yeast, molds), many have very exact criteria for when they throw out showers of billions of spores. For example, Cladosporium will produce showers of billions of spores, preferably around noon. Whereas Sporobolomyces will produce showers around midnight. Therefore, it is important to culture an environment when the symptoms are the worst. For example, an asthmatic who awakens at 3 a.m. should have his bedroom cultured at that time, not at 10 in the morning when he is off at school or work.

Rogers SA, A Thirteen Month Work, Leisure, Sleep Environmental Fungal Survey, ANN ALLERGY, 52, 338-341, May 1984.

ALLERGY TO POLLEN, DUST, MITES, AND MOLDS

Pollens, dust, mites and molds are standard common anti-gens tested by nearly all allergists. However, extensive research has been done over the last few years that has shown that many other fungi are present in the environment that are not being tested for. Other studies demonstrate that when these fungi are tested and found to be positive and used in treatment, that remarkable improvements occur in various conditions that were resistant to prior treatment. Mold sensitivities can even mimic chemical sensitivity symptoms.

Furthermore, it turns out that the target organ for mold sensitivity does not have to be limited to a runny nose or eczema. Likewise, mold sensitivity can cause brain symptoms such as inability to concentrate, fatigue, depression and other organ systems can be targets for this sensitivity.

Sheldon JM, Lovell RG, Matthews KP, A MANUAL OF CLINICAL ALLERGY, W.B. Saunders Co., Philadelphia, 1967.

Mold allergy has historically caused just about any symptom and can even mimic the sick building syndrome (also called the tight building syndrome). In cases where it is assumed that chemical sensitivity is the cause of symptoms, often mold allergy has been found to be the actual culprit.

Rogers SA, A practical approach to the person with suspected indoor air quality problems, INTERNATIONAL CLINICAL NUTRITION REVIEWS 11:3, 126-130, July 1991.

Mold allergy, of course, is well-known as one of the ubiquitous contributors to chronic rhinitis, otitis, headaches, migraines, asthma, bronchitis, recurrent upper respiratory infections, eczema, fatigue and much more.

Hyposensitization to mold to which the patient is sensitive on testing, fosters the development of blocking antibodies to "turn off" or at least down regulate mold-induced symptoms.

Al-Doory Y, Domson J, MOLD ALLERGY, Philadelphia, Lee & Febiger, 1984.

Dreborg S, Agrell B, Foucard T. et al. A double -blind, multicenter immunotherapy trial in children, using a purified and standardized Cladosporium herbarbum preparation. I. Clinical results. ALLERGY 1986; 41: 131-140

Rogers SA, A Thirteenth Month Work, Leisure, Sleep Environmental Fungal Survey, ANN ALLERGY, 52, 338-341, May 1984.

Rogers SA, Resistant Cases, Response to Mold Immunotherapy and Environmental and Dietary Controls, CLINICAL ECOLOGY, ARCHIVES FOR HUMAN ECOLOGY IN HEALTH AND DISEASE, 5, 3, 115- 120, 1987/1988.

Rogers SA, A comparison of commercially available mold Survey Services, ANN ALLERGY, 50, 37-40, January, 1983.

Rogers SA, In-home Fungal Studies, Methods to Increase the Yield, ANN ALLERGY, 49, 35-37, July, 1982.

TESTING

SERIAL DILUTION ENDPOINT TITRATION

Traditionally, allergists have tested patients with one or a few strengths of an antigen and used this as an all or nothing determination of whether or not a patient was sensitive to the antigen. Then the dose arbitrarily was raised with each injection until a cutoff point was determined. Sometimes this cutoff point was determined by severe reaction or death of the patient. It therefore has made much more sense to find the top tolerated dose for each antigen within the safety of the allergist's office and not turn the patient loose on an unsuspecting pediatrician or family physician who is giving the injections.

Editorial, Systemic reactions from allergen immunotherapy, J ALLER CLIN IMMUNOL, 567, May 1992.

When dealing with potentially lethal substances (which all injectible antigens are), it is not only scientific fact but common sense to determine the safest and most effective dose for each individual antigen within the safety of the allergist's office. Then release him to have his injections given when there is a marked decrease in the probability of possibly fatal reactions.

Titration merely means testing with several strengths to find the very best or optimum (and safest) dose. This is common sense even to non-allergists and non-physicians. Rather than testing everyone to one or two dose strengths and blindly raising the dose with each injection, it makes more sense and has been proven to be safer to find the optimum dose of each antigen in each patient who receives it. It does not make the erroneous and dangerous assumption that you are just as allergic to dust as I am, for example.

Also, in this way the optimum dose is found for each particular antigen and the erroneous assumption is not made that one individual is just as sensitive to one antigen as he is to another, which would be equally absurd.

The JOURNAL OF THE AMERICAN MEDICAL ASSOCI-ATION (vol. 28, no. 10, September 11, 1987) presents an article by the Council on Scientific Affairs, p. 1365:

"**Skin test endpoint titration provides a useful and effective measure of patient sensitivity.** Controlled studies have shown that the intradermal method of skin test endpoint **titration is effective for quantifying sensitivity** to ragweed pollen extract and for identifying patients highly sensitive to ragweed. This method provides reliability comparable to that of in vitro leukocyte histamine release and radio allergosorbent test. Controlled studies have shown that the prick test method of skin test endpoint titration can be used as a measure of response to immunotherapy with cat extract."

Furthermore, skin endpoint titration has been successfully used for decades by thousands of allergists and ENT physicians and there are no published papers of fatalities using this method, but there are published papers of fatalities using the traditional non-individualized or "canned" method.

The American Medical Association and the American Academy of Allergy and Immunology have found it important to use this technique with highly dangerous antigens such as hymenoptera (stinging insects like bees, wasps, hornets and yellow jackets) and cat antigens.

The reason ragweed or cat antigens were used as an example in these studies is because they are unique antigens.

Ragweed has a very precise or well-defined season and limited cross - antigenicity, while exposure to cats can be controlled.

Van Metre TE, Marsh DG, Adkinson NF, Kagey-Sobotki A, Khattignavong A, Norman PS, Rosenberg GL. Immunotherapy for cat asthma. J ALLERCLIN IMMUNOL 1988;6:1055-1068.

Furthermore, the American Academy of Allergy and Immunology Training Program Director's Committee published "unproven techniques" but it did not include serial dilution titration:

AAAI Training Program Director's Committee Report. Topics related to controversial practices that should be taught in an allergy and immunology training program. J ALLERCLIN IMMUNOL 1994;93:955-66.

There are no papers at this point in time to refute serial dilution endpoint titration that do not have errors in their methodology. However, there are scores of papers showing the benefits of this technique. As well, this is the very foundation of all scientific research: to find the optimal dose of each substance given to each individual organism.

The last point, but one of the most important evidences for SDET, is that of the perfect mathematical progression of wheal size (skin reactivity) that reflects precise and direct immune system involvement. For with every 5-fold increase in test dose strength, there is a 2 mm. increase in skin reactivity. This precise and reproducible occurrence reflects the absolute dose and immune system relationship.

So SDET is the antithesis of experimental, for it is currently the most precise in vivo quantitation of the body's immune system that can be easily, safely, and inexpensively performed in the physician's office. It is clear that the canned conventional "one dose for all" technique is potentially more dangerous (as has been born out in studies) and less accurate and less scientific.

IMMUNOTHERAPY WITHOUT TITRATION CAN BE DANGEROUS

It is evident the technique of SDET for individualized, titrated, or tailor-made extracts is more scientific and far safer for the patient. There are no published studies connecting the disease polyateritis nodosa with SDET. But 6 of 20 consecutive patients with the disease had the onset of vasculitic symptoms coincide with hyposensitization therapy that was not titrated.

Phanuphal P, Kohler PF, Onset of polyarteritis nodosa during allergic hyposensitization treatment. AMER J MED, 68, 479-485, April 1980.

Likewise finding the top tolerated doses within the safety of the allergist's office as with SDET makes more sense than to arbitrarily raise the dose of every antigen at each injection. In fact in a large medical school, adverse reactions to injections were seen in 51% of patients. And 77% of these reactions were seen on increasing doses. So **in 10 years (1977-1987) over a quarter of the patients reacted when doses were raised when non-titrated extracts were used.** This is foolish when there is a time-tested and more accurate and scientific method:

Weber RW, Vaughn TR, Dolen WK. A ten year review of adverse reactions to immunotherapy. J ALLERGY CLIN IMMUNOL, abs. #510 p 295, Jan 1988

Some have argued that titrated doses are too low to be effective, but studies have disproven this as well. In fact even giving them sublingually relieved the symptoms in 72% of patients. And when they were given nasal provocation tests with the antigen after treatment, their resistance to getting symptoms was in some cases up to a 1000-fold higher:

Scadding GK, Brostoff J, Low dose sublingual therapy in patients with allergic rhinitis due to house dust mite. CLIN ALLERGY, 1986, 16: 483-491.

As well, scientists have proven this in rats:
Shellam GR, Nossal GJV, mechanism of induction of immunological tolerance. IV. The effects of ultra-low doses of flagellin. IMMUNOLOGY, 1968, 14: 273-284.

Other researchers have confirmed that conventional or standard immunotherapy **without titration** has been so risky that "when these potent extracts were used, allergen injections initially **resulted in a greater number of systemic reactions."**

Bonsquet J, Michel FB, Specific immunotherapy for asthma: Is it effective? J ALLERGY CLIN IMMUNOL 94:1, 1-11, 1994.

Locky RF, Benedict LM, Turkeltaub PC, Bilkantz SC, fatalities from immunotherapy & skin testing. J ALLERGY CLIN IMMUNOL 79:660-77, 1987

Immunotherapy fosters the production of IgG blocking antibody, and symptoms gradually lessen and often dissapear entirely. But to merely treat symptoms with drugs is to invite further problems in other target organs. For example, prescribed **antihistamines can trigger poten-**

tially fatal cardiac arrhythmias, compromise the xenobiotic detoxification system and inhibit the potassium pump in the heart muscle cells!

Good AP, Rochwood R, Schad P, Loratadine and ventricular tachycardia. AMER J CARDIOL 74:207-209, 1994.

As demonstrated in the Laboratory section, to use drugs to mask symptoms merely hastens the possibility of disaster in a different and unexpected area of the body. The problem is that a physician in a different area of specialization is consulted and none suspect the actual cause if they are from drug-oriented, non biochemically trained medicine.

We could continue this treatise indefinitely on the adverse effect of taking medications. The Canadian researcher Dr. Lorne J Brandes published his findings in the May 1994 JOURNAL OF THE NATIONAL CANCER INSTITUTE: Several **antihistamines** like Hismanil, Clariten, and Atarax **promote cancer growth, even in low doses.**
So no insurance company has a scientific basis on which to reject titrated allergen testing. For remember, the **JOURNAL OF THE AMERICAN MEDICAL ASSOCIATION's** (Vol. 28, no.10, September 11, 1987) article by the Council on Scientific Affairs, Pg. 1365:

"Skin test endpoint titration provides a useful and effective measure of patient sensitivity. Controlled studies have shown that the intradermal method of skin test endpoint titration **is effective for quantifying sensitivity."**

Another very important reason for titrating patients is that allergen extracts at this point in time are not reliably standardized. Small variations could kill a very sensitive patient.

41

"Results indicate that standardized and conventional extracts are frequently similar but are not directly interchangeable." This quote is from:

Lavins BJ, Dolen WK, Nelson HS, Weber RW. Use of standardized and conventional allergen extracts in prick-skin testing. J ALLER AND CLIN IMMUNOL 1992;89:658-66.
Likewise, the histamine content of commercial antigens from four commercial sources was measured and found to be variable. The conclusion was "histamine found in some allergen extracts could, under extreme circumstances, produce false positive results in skin testing and in basophil histamine-release assays and could affect the result of research that uses intact pollens or allergen extracts." Well, what about the patient? It could also cause false positives and this is another reason for being careful to determine whether the degree of sensitivity is clinically significant as well as to determine a safe enough dose of the antigen if it is required.

Williams PB, Nolte H, Dolen WK, Coepke JW, Selner JC. The histamine content of allergen extracts. J ALLER CLIN IMMUNOL 1992;89:738-45.

Oral Hyposensitization

Extracts can also be given orally as many references in the SDET section will show. It is obvious nowadays, that drugs and antigens can be absorbed not only across the lung membranes (inhaled asthma drugs), and the skin (estrogen, nicotine, nitroglycerine and motion sickness patches). The nasal and oral routes are also used for drugs (nitroglycerin, ergotamine) and antigens.

Giovane A, et al, A three-year double-blind placebo-controlled study with specific oral immunotherapy to Dermataphagoides: evidence of safety and efficacy in paediatric patients. CLIN AND EXPER ALLERGY, 1994: 74 (Jan): 53-59

PUBLICATIONS SUPPORTING
THE SCIENTIFIC VALIDITY SDET.

This technique has been done for over a half a century and is currently used by over 2000 physicians. And a review of the scientific literature shows it is safer and more scientific, as explained earlier.

Council on Scientific Affairs. In vivo diagnostic testing and immunotherapy for allergy. Report I, part I, part II, Report II of the Allergy Panel. JAMA 258:10;1363, Sept. 11, 1987.

Mabry RL. Skin endpoint titration: history, theory, and practice. Dist. by Meridian Biomedical Inc., 1700 Royston Lane, Round Rock, TX 78664 (an FDA-approved allergy laboratory, which produces extracts).

Williams RI. Skin titration: testing and treatment. OTOLARYNGOL CLIN OF N AMERICA 1971;4:3.

Williams RI. Technique of serial dilution antigen titration. ARCH OTOLARYNGOL 1969;89:109.

Willoughby JW. Serial dilution titration skin tests in inhalant allergy: a clinical quantitative assessment of biologic skin reactivity to allergenic extracts. OTOLARYNGOL CLIN OF N AMERICA 1974;7:579.

Willoughby JW. Diagnosis of allergy by serial dilution skin end-point titration. CONTINUING EDUCATION FOR FAMILY PHYSICIANS 1979;11(3):21.

Willoughby JW. Intracutaneous serial dilution titration in clinical allergy. Printed privately for the postgraduate course in clinical allergy, April 1973, Kansas City, MO, available from American Academy of Otolaryngic Allergy, Silver Springs, MD.

Rocklin RE, Sheffer AL, Greinedeker DK, Melmon KL. Generation of antigen-specific suppressor cells during allergy desensitization. NEJM 1976;30:1378-85.

Ali M, Ramanarayana MP, Nalebuff DJ, Fadal RG, Willoughby JW. Serum concentration of allergen specific IgG antibody in inhalant allergens; effect of specific immunotherapy. AM J CLIN PATH 1983;80:290.

Rinkel HJ. Inhalant allergy, part I: the whealing response of the skin to serial dilution testing. ANN ALLERGY 1949;7:625-30,650.

Rinkel HJ. The management of clinical allergy. ARCH OTOLARYNGOL 1963;77:50.

Rinkel HJ. The management of clinical allergy, part II: etiologic factors and skin titration. ARCH OTOLARYNGOL 1963;7:42.

Rogers SA. Resistant cases: response to mold immunotherapy and environmental and dietary controls. CLIN ECOLOGY 1987/8;3(V):115-20.

Van Niekerk CH, DeWet JI. Efficacy of grass-maize pollen oral immunotherapy in patients with seasonal hay fever: a double-blind study. CLIN ALLERGY 1987;17:507-13.

Mandell M, Conte A. A role of allergy in arthritis, rheumatism and polysymptomatic cerebral, visceral and somatic disorders: a double-blind study. J INTERNAT ACAD PREVENT MED 1982, VOL. 7;2:5-16.

Turkelaub PC, Rastogi SC, Baer H, Anderson MC, Norman PS. A standardized quantitative skin-test assay of allergen potency and stability: Studies on the allergen dose-response curve and effect of wheat, erythema, and patient selection on assay results. J ALLERGY IMMUNOL 70: 343-52, 1982

In Addition

"Skin testing is the most widely used in vivo method of standardizing allergy extracts", and "skin testing is the most clinically relevant measure of the potency of an allergen extract, and no specialized or expensive equipment is necessary". (ANN ALLERGY, p 108, Jan 1991).

Furthermore, studies using 4 commercial skin test devices that are commonly used by allergists who do not titrate showed there was no standard agreement, ie. "the four devices do not give comparable skin reactions". Therefore they are not only inaccurate, but dangerous:

Ryhal B7, Halpern GM, Davis PA, Garcelon M, Gershwin ME, A Comparison of four prick skin test devices in patient with allergic rhinitis, IMMUNOL & ALLERGY PRACT XIII:9, 353/11 - 353/16, Sept. 1991

The U.S. government National Institutes of Allergy and Infectious Diseases stated that "Standardized allergens should be made available in forms permitting dilution or multiple dose forms so that dose-response relationships can be established":

Proceedings of the task force on guidelines for standardizing old and new technologies used for the diagnosis and treatment of allergic diseases, J ALLERGY CLIN IMMUNOL, 82:3, part2, 1988.

And Johns Hopkins researchers demonstrated that in highly sensitive asthmatic patients, using intradermal skin-test end point titration for immunotherapy "was well tolerated, significantly decreased skin and bronchial responses to cat extract, and significantly increased IgG antibodies to cat extract":

Van Metre TE, Marsh DG, Adkenson NF, Sobotka AK, Khattignavong A, Norman PS, Rosenburg GL, Immunotherapy for cat asthma, J ALLERGY CLIN IMMUNOL, 82: 6, 1055-1068, 1988.

FOOD ALLERGY

Food Allergy Can Mimic Any Symptom

Food allergy is a known cause for multiple hidden symptoms. In fact it is unusual to find a patient with resistant rhinitis, migraines, asthma, recurrent infections, fatigue, colitis, arthritis, depression, chemical sensitivity, and many other resistant symptoms who does not have one or more foods that can exacerbate the symptoms. This allergy does not need to be restricted to IgE or IgG mediated sensitivities, for there are a dozen mechanisms by which foods can cause symptoms: and diet trials are the least expensive way to diagnose many.

Brostoff J, Challacombe SJ, FOOD ALLERGY AND INTOLERANCE, Bailliere Tindall, Phill., 1987

One of the more common problems food allergies can cause are middle ear fluid in young children with recurrent infections and hearing loss. A common way of treating this is with tympanostomy tubes, otherwise known as PE (polyethylene pressure-equalizing) tubes, but these tubes can actually cause hearing loss, not to mention the remote possibility of anesthetic death. It makes more sense to identify the hidden food sensitivities that most often cause this ear fluid and these symptoms and eliminate them.

Scheck A. Tympanostomy tubes may cause hearing loss. FAMILY PRACTICE NEWS 1993(3/15);3:24.

Green RG. Diet and otitis media. CANADIAN FAMILY PHYSICIAN 1983(Jan);29:15.

Furthermore, food allergy can go on to cause part or all of many other symptoms, such as asthma.

Rowe AH, Young EJ. Bronchial asthma due to food allergy alone in 95 patients. JAMA 1959;169:1158.

Hoj L, Osterballe O, Bundgaard B, Weeke B, Weiss M. A double-blind controlled trial of elemental diet in severe perennial asthma. ALLERGY 1981;36:257.

Ogle KA, Bullock JD. Children with allergic rhinitis and/or bronchial asthma treated with elimination diet: a five year follow-up. ANN ALLERGY 1980;44:273.

Indeed, food allergy can cause any symptom you can think of, from asthma, bronchitis, emphysema, chronic rhinitis, Meniere's disease, chronic interstitial cystitis marked by unsuccessful treatment by 2 or more competent urologists, as well as nephrotic syndrome, migraines, epilepsy, arthritis and many other disorders.

Panush RS, Carter RL, Katz P, et al, Diet Therapy for rheumatoid arthritis,ARTHRITIS & RHEUMATISM 26:4; 462-470, 1983

Ogle KA, Bullock JD. Children with allergic rhinitis and/or bronchial asthma treated with elimination diet. ANN ALLERGY 1977;39:8.

Rowe AH, Rowe A. Food allergy: its role in emphysema and chronic bronchitis. DIS CHEST 1965;48:609.

Derlacki EL. Food sensitization as a cause of perennial nasal allergy. ANN ALLERGY 1955;13:682.

Sampson HA, et al, Fatal and near-fatal anaphylactic reactions to food in children and adolescents. NEJM 1992; 327:380-4.

Davison HM. The role of food sensitivity in nasal allergy. ANN ALLERGY 1951;9:568.

Piness G, Miller H. The importance of food sensitization in allergic rhinitis. J ALLERGY 1931;2:73.

Rowe AH, Rowe A Jr. Perennial nasal allergy due to food sensitization. J ASTHMA RES 1965;3:141.

Endicott JN, Stucker FJ. Allergy in Meniere's disease related to fluctuating hearing loss. Preliminary findings in a double-blind crossover clinical study. LARYNGOSCOPE 1977;87:1650.

Powell NB, Powell EB, Thomas OC, Queng JT, McGovern JP. Allergy of the lower urinary tract. J UROL 1972;107:631-634.

Pastinszky I. The allergic diseases of the male genitourinary tract with special reference to allergic urethritis and cystitis. UROL INT 1959;9:288-305.

Sandberg DH, McIntosh RM, Bernstein CW, Carr R, Strauss J. Severe steroid-responsive nephrosis associated with hypersensitivity. LANCET 1977;1:388.

Law-Chin-Yung L, Freed DLJ. Nephrotic syndrome due to milk allergy. LANCET 1977;1:1056.

Monro J, Carini C, Brostoff J, Zilkha K. Food allergy in migraine: study of dietary exclusion and RAST. LANCET 1980;2:1.

Egger J, Wilson J, Carter CM, Turner MW, Soothill JF. Is migraine food allergy? A double-blind controlled trial of oligoantigenic diet treatment. LANCET 1983;2:865.

Dees SC. Allergic epilepsy. ANN ALLERGY 1951;9:446.

Adamson WB, Sellers ED. Observations on the incidence of the hypersensitive state in one hundred cases of epilepsy. J ALLERGY 1933;5:315.

Fein BT, Kamin PB. Allergy, convulsive disorders and epilepsy. ANN ALLERGY 1968;26:241.

Panush RS: Food induced (allergic) arthritis. Clinical and serological slides. J RHEUMATOL 17:591-94, 1990

Felder M, de Blecourt ACE, Wuthrich B: Food allergy in patients with rheumatoid arthritis. CLIN RHEUMATOL 6: 181-84, 1987

Campbell MB. Neurologic manifestations of allergic disease. ANN ALLERGY 1973;31:485.

Van de Loar MAFJ, Van der Korst JK: Rheumatoid Arthritis, Food and allergy. SEMINARS ARTH RHEUM 21: 12-23, 1991

Karjalainen J, et al. A bovine albumin peptide as a possible trigger of insulin-dependent diabetes mellitus. NEJM, July 30, 1992, 302-307.

Maclarren N, Atkinson M. Is insulin-dependent diabetes mellitus environmentally induced? NEJM 1992; 327:348-9

Kjeldsen-Kragh J, et al, Controlled trial of fasting and one-year vegetarian diet in rheumatoid arthritis. LANCET 1991; 338:899-900.

DIAGNOSTIC DIETS

Elimination diets have been invaluable in the diagnosis and treatment of food allergy and various diets require a great deal of instruction and patient education and time. Therefore, it is often less expensive and more efficacious to give the patients books in addition to counseling in the office.

Organic foods are often necessary as studies have shown that organic foods have up to as much as 2 1/2 times the nutrient value of foods grown on commercial soils that have become depleted:

Smith R, Organic foods versus supermarket foods. J APP NUTR 45:1, 35-39, 1993

Many books spell out the diets for patients and are a necessary adjunct to treatment, since patient education and responsibility are a hallmark of non-drug-oriented medicine.

Rapp, DJ, IS THIS YOUR CHILD? WM Morrow and Co, 1991

Rogers SA, THE E.I. SYNDROME, Prestige Publishing, Syracuse NY, 1986

Mandell M. THE 5-DAY ALLERGY RELIEF SYSTEM

Randolph T, Moss R, AN ALTERNATIVE APPROACH TO ALLERGIES, Bantam Books, NY, 1987

MACROBIOTIC DIETS

Some conditions are so severe that exceedingly strict diets are needed for a temporary amount of time in order to bring about wellness. One of the most strict diets is the macrobiotic diet which has increased cancer survival against all odds. In fact it more than triples survival. In the **JOURNAL OF THE AMERICAN COLLEGE OF NUTRITION** Carter and his medical school epidemilogic team have shown how the macrobiotic diet can more than triple cancer survival. If men do all that medicine has to offer for cancer of the prostate (chemotherapy, surgery, hormones, radiation, etc.), as one example, the median survival is **six** years. If, however, they do not do this, and save tens of thousands of dollars, but instead do the macrobiotic diet for a minimum of three months, median survival goes up from **6 years to 19 years.** In other words **the macrobiotic diet can more than triple the survival** compared with expensive high tech medicine.

Likewise, they showed marked increases in survival in other types of cancers, such as cancer of the pancreas, which has a very poor record in general medicine.

If you do everything medicine has to offer, in one year 10% are still alive. If they do the macrobiotic diet, in one year 52% are alive. The survival is more than 5-fold. There is no contest:

Carter JP, Saxe GP, Newbold V, Peres CE, Campbell RJ, Bernal-Green, Dietary management may improve survival from nutritionally-linked cancers based on analysis of representative cases. J AMER COLL NUTR 12:3, 209-226, 1993

Needless to say, the diet has also improved many people with multiple chemical sensitivities, asthma, eczema, chronic sinusitis, and many undiagnosable conditions or conditions that are considered to be "end of the road" for which nothing more can be done.

Likewise,"DR. DEAN ORNISH'S PROGRAM FOR REVERSING HEART DISEASE" (Ornish D, Random House NY, 1990) has been equally successful when everything else that medicine has to offer has failed. This is a relaxed version of the macrobiotic diet. They used people who had endstage coronary artery disease who had had bypass surgery and cholesterol-lowering drugs and were still clotting off new vessels. They instead stopped everything and went on the diet program and actually reversed the arteriosclerotic lesions on the PET scans within a year and markedly reduced their symptoms (Ornish 1990, LANCET). In other words, they too, accomplished with a diet what high tech medicine failed to do.

There are many books that are recommend to patients that explain the various elimination and macrobiotic diets (also see books in FOOD ALLERGY section). Some of the books to explain this macrobiotic diet and its unprecendented success rate against all odds are:

East West Foundation, Cancer-Fee, 30 WHO TRIUMPHED OVER CANCER NATURALLY, Japan Publ., NY, 1991.

Ornish D, DR DEAN ORNISH'S PROGRAM FOR REVERSING HEART DISEASE, Random House, NY 1990

Rogers SA YOU ARE WHAT YOU ATE, Prestige Publ, Syracuse NY, 1991

Rogers SA, THE CURE IS IN THE KITCHEN, Prestige Publ, Syracuse NY 1992

Gallinger S, Rogers SA, MACRO MELLOW, Prestige Publ, Syracuse NY,1993

There are , of course, hundreds of papers on the chemical constituents of macrobiotic foods, called phytochemicals. It has been known for decades that many phytochemicals have strong anti-carcinogenic effects, not only for prevention, but also to reverse cancers once they have begun to grow. That data is far too voluminous for this monograph.

Anderson KE, Kappas A, Dietary regulation of cytochrome P450, ANN REV NUTR,11: 141-67, 1991

Yuesheng 2, Tallaloy p, et al, A major inducer of anticarcinogenic protective enzymes from broccoli. Isolation and elucidation of structure. PROC NAT ACAD SCI 89:2399- 2403, 1992

Last, the dietary recommendations of every national health organization over the last decade has been slowly inching toward the principles of the macrobiotic diet (more grains, greens, and beans, fruits and vegetables; fewer meats, sweets, fat, salt and alcohol). There is no organization refuting these recommendations. But I say "inching", because the U.S. government has just recommended lowering the daily fat content of the diet to 30%! But it is only when it is 5% that healing and reversal of arteriosclerotic lesions and cancers occur.

Food Allergy Injections

This technique is similar to the SEDT or serial endpoint dilution titration techniques, but instead of testing several antigens at once, only one needle is tested at a time. As a result, this technique can provoke symptoms and has been called the provocation-neutralization technique. This is because once the symptom is provoked or turned on, often you can go to the next lower dose and turn it off or neutralize it. However, a symptom does not necessarily always have to be provoked with this technique.

Regardless of whether a symptoms is provoked or not, this also uses 5-fold dilutions to titrate for the safest and optimally tolerated dose. It is a useful way to find the exact treatment dose to put in the vial to administer. Testing and treating food allergies has been efficacious for people whose food sensitivities are not controlled with diets alone.

King WP, Rubin WA, Fadal RG, Ward WA, Trevino RJ, Pierce WB, Stewart WA, Boyles JH. Provocation/neutralization: a two- part study, part I. The intracutaneous provocative food test: a multi-center comparison study OTOLARYNGOLOGY HEAD AND NECK SURGERY 1988(Sept);99(3):263-72.

King WP, Rubin WA, Fadal RG, Ward WA, Trevino RJ, Pierce WB, Stewart WA, Boyles JH. Provocation/neutralization: a two- part study, part II. Subcutaneous neutralization therapy: a multi-center study. OTOLARYNGOLOGY HEAD AND NECK SURGERY 1988(Sept.);99(3):272-278.

Also see all references for SDET and P-N

Hormones

Thyroid deficiency is a commonly understood medical condition and cause of fatigue. However, in a world where chemicals are triggering people to make more antibodies, thyroid autoantibodies should be checked whenever there is a problem with the thyroid. Of course, thyroid deficiency can exacerbate chronic rhinitis, asthma, constipation and irritable bowel symptoms, fatigue, toxic encephalopathy, and the symptoms of multiple chemical sensitivity.

Likewise, the adrenal or stress gland can be hypo-functioning due to many causes. Pesticides can also damage glands and nutrient deficiencies can impair their function. (see reference in Pesticide Section). In fatigue cases, it is particularly important to look for the lazy adrenal by doing a cortrosyn stimulation test and an unconjugated DHEA.

Withers BT. Hypometabolism in allergy: a review for otolaryngologists. LARYNGOSCOPE 1974;84:43.

Hollander AR. Hypometabolism in relation to ear, nose, and throat disorders.
ARCHIVES OF OTOLARYNGOLOGY 1956;63:135.

Jeffries W. SAFE USES OF HYDROCORTISONE, Charles C. Thomas Co., Springfield, FL, 1981

PROVOCATION-NEUTRALIZATION
PHENOL

Phenol(hydroxybenzene or carbonic acid) is a standard preservative in allergy extracts. However, not everyone who could benefit from extracts is able to tolerate phenol. Some are sensitive to the very preservative in the extracts that they require.

Skea D, McAvoy D, Broder L, Phenol amplifies complement-fixing activity and induces IgG-precipitating activity in grain-dust extract. J ALLERGY CLIN IMMUNOL 1988; 81: 557-63

LaVia MF, LaVia DS, Phenol derivatives are immunosuppressive in mice. DRUG AND CHEM TOXICOL 2 (1/2): 167-177, 1979

Deichmann WB, Keplinger ML, Phenols and phenolic compounds, PATTY'S INDUSTRIAL HYGIENE AND TOXICOLOGY, Patty FA, John Wiley and sons, NY, p2567-2627, 1981
Nour-Eldin F, Preliminary report: Uptake of phenol by vascular and brain tissue, MICROVASCULAR RES 2, 224-225, 1970

PROVOCATION-NEUTRALIZATION IS USED TO DIAGNOSE FOOD AND CHEMICAL SENSITIVITIES

Since the provocation-neutralization technique is very useful in diagnosing chemical sensitivity and since phenol and/or glycerine sensitivity is very common in chemically sensitive people, it is imperative to test them to these antigens to see if they can tolerate the actual preservatives and stabilizers used in injections. The toxic and procarcinogenic effects of phenol can be found in any general toxicology text.

Phenol sensitivity was first thought of when people reacted to injections even though they were titrated. When this preservative was omitted, they did fine. But a method to test it was needed that could be performed in the office single-blind or double-blind to rule out malingering. The provocation-neutralization test has filled this need for over a quarter of a century, with no published adverse outcomes of the technique. In fact it saves lives, as reactions discovered in an office setting are much more safely treated than out of the office.

Even the United States government's National Institutes of Health own medical journal in 1987 published the provocation-neutralization technique for testing for adverse reactions to chemicals. Furthermore, the EPA also listed this technique in it's INDOOR AIR REFERENCE BIBLIOGRAPHY, July 1989.

Rogers, Diagnosing the Tight Building Syndrome, ENVIRONMENTAL HEALTH PERSPECTIVES, 76, 195-198, 1987.

In addition, provocation-neutralization (P-N) has been successfully used for decades by thousands of allergists and ENT physicians and there are no published papers of fatalities using this method. But there are published papers of fatalities using the traditional non-individualized method. P-N has been successfully used to test foods and chemicals for well over a quarter of a century.

Provocation-neutralization is a similar technique to skin endpoint titration. The only difference is you only test one antigen at a time. Often, but not always, a symptom can be provoked or triggered by the "wrong" dose and then turned off or neutralized by the "correct" dose. Hence the name of the technique, provocation-neutralization.

It is ironic that the American Medical Association and the American Academy of Allergy and Immunology have found it important to use the end-point titration technique with highly dangerous antigens such as hymenoptera(stinging insects) and cat antigens, but have gone on record as being opposed to provocation/neutralization in general.

The American Academy of Allergy and Immunology Training Program Director's Committee listed under "unproven techniques" the provocation-neutralization method. But it did not include serial dilution titration, which is a similar technique and that they use. Their only, **solo evidence** for not using the provocation-neutralization technique was the study by Jewett. This is the only paper they site as as excuse to invalidate the technique.

But this solo paper that they hang their decision on is frought with 13 errors, the most flagrant of which is **they had the technique backwards**. On line 6 of the paper, under "Procedures", they explicately describe the treatment dose as "that doses that grows 2mm in wheal diameter". Actually, that is the perfect description of the dose that turns on or provokes symptoms. It is not the treatment dose.

So no wonder that their conclusion at the end of the study was that the technique does not work! Of course it doesn't work: they had it absolutely backwards! **The dose they were using to try to turn off symptoms is the actual dose that turns on or provokes symptoms.** So, of course, they could not turn off a single symptom because they were using the perfect dose with which to turn them on, if they were provokable.

This was a non-peer-reviewed paper full of 13 errors and failed to prove anything except that the people who did the study had inadequate knowledge of the technique. Since that is the only reason for rejecting provocation-neutralization (P-N), that reason would not hold up in any court of law.

Unfortunately, other groups, assuming that the AAAI knew what they were doing, then based their critique of P-N on the recommendation of the AAAI, not on scientific fact. They did not investigate the facts for themselves and merely "followed the lead" and likewise inappropriately black-balled this technique.

AAAI Training Program Director's Committee Report. Topics related to controversial practices that should be taught in an allergy and immunology training program. JOURNAL OF ALLERGY AND CLINICAL IMMUNOLOGY 1994; 93:955-66.

Jewett DL, Fein G. Greenberg MH. A double blind study of symptom provocation to determine food sensitivity. N ENG J MED 1990;323:429-33.

United States Environmental Protection Agency, INDOOR

AIR REFERENCED BIBLIOGRAPHY, Office of Health and Environmental Assessment, Washington, D.C., July, 1990, pg. C81 and C162. (The provocation/neutralization test was cited here under methods to diagnosis chemical sensitivity.)

The P/N technique also was published in ENVIRONMENT INTERNATIONAL, a journal that goes to 152 countries:
Rogers SA, Indoor Fungi as Part of the Cause of Recalcitrant Symptoms of the Tight Building Syndrome, ENVIRONMENT INTERNATIONAL 17,4,271-276, 1991.

The provocation-neutralization technique has also been published in numerous other peer-reviewed journals. Also it is the only technique for diagnosing chemical sensitivity that was featured in 5 major landmark international indoor symposia:

Rogers SA, A Practical Approach to the Person With Suspected Indoor Air Quality Problems, THE 5TH QUALITY CONFERENCE ON INDOOR AIR QUALITY AND CLIMATE,Toronto, Canada, Canada Mortage and Housing Corporation, Ottawa, Ontario, volume 5, 345-349, 1990.

Rogers SA, Diagnosing the Tight Building Syndrome, an intradermal method to provoke chemically induced symptoms, MAN AND HIS ECOSYSTEM, PROCEEDINGS OF THE 8TH WORLD CLEAN AIR CONGRESS 1989, Brasser, LJ, Mulder, WC, editors. The Hague, Netherlands, Society for Clean Air in The Netherlands, P.O. Box 186, 2600 AD Delft, The Nethlands. 199-204, volume 1, 1989.

Rogers SA, Diagnosing the Tight Building Syndrome, an intradermal method to provoke chemically induced symptoms, HEALTHY BUILDINGS '88, CIB conference in

Stockholm, Sweden, September, 1988, Swedish Council for Building Research, Stockholm Sweden, Berlund, B, Lindvall, T, Mansson, L-G, editors, 371, 1988

Rogers SA, Diagnosing the Tight Building Syndrome, Indoor Air '87, PROCEEDINGS OF THE 4TH INTERNATIONAL CONFERENCE ON INDOOR AIR QUALITY AND CLIMATE, West Berlin, Seifert, B, Esdorn, H, Fischer, M, Ruden, H, Wegner, J, editors, Institute for Water, Soil and Air Hygiene, D 1000 Berlin 33, volume 2, 772-776, August, 1987.

Rogers SA, Indoor Air Quality and Environmentally Induced Illness, A technique to revoke chemically induced symptoms in patients. PROCEEDINGS OF THE ASHRAE CONFERENCE, IAQ 86, Managing Indoor Air for Health and Energy conservation, 71- 77, ASHRAE, 1791 Tullie Circle, NE, Atlanta, GA 30329

PEER REVIEWED SCIENTIFIC STUDIES
SUPPORTING P-N FOR TESTING.

Boris M, et al. "Late phase response treated with neutralization therapy", presented to the 21st Scientific Session of the American Academy of Environmental Medicine, October 31, 1987, Nashville, Tennessee.

Brostoff J, Scadding G. Low dose sublingual therapy in patients with allergic rhinitis due to house dust mite. CLINICAL ALLERGY 1986;16:483-91.

Brostoff J, "A double-blind crossover placebo-controlled study of neutralization", presented to the 20th Advance Seminar of the American Academy of Environmental Medicine, October 27, 1986, Clearwater, Florida.

Boris M, Schiff M, Weindorf S. Antigen-induced asthma attenuated by neutralization therapy. CLINICAL ECOLOGY 1985;3:59-62.

Boris MN, Schiff M, Weindorf S. Injection of low-dose antigen attenuates the response to subsequent bronchoprovocative challenge. OTOLARYNG HEAD NECK SURG 1988;98:539-545.

Draper WL. Food testing in allergy. ARCH OTOLARYNGOL 1972;95:169-171.

King WP, Rubin WA, Fadal RG, Ward WA, Trevion RJ, Pierce WB, Stewart WA, Boyles JH. Provocation-neutralization: a two- part study, part I. The intracutaneous provocative food test: a multi-center comparison study. OTOLARYNGOL HEAD NECK SURG 1988;99(3):263-272.

King WP, Fadal R, Ward W, Trevion R, Pierce W, Stewart

J, Boyles JH. Provocation-neutralization: a two-part study, part II. Subcutaneous neutralization therapy: a multi-center study. OTOLARYNGOL HEAD NECK SURG 1988;99(3):272-8.

Lee LK, Kniker WT, Campos T. Aggressive coseasonal immunotherapy in mountain cedar pollen allergy. ARCH OTOLARYNGOL 1982;108:782.

Lee CH, et al. Provocative testing and treatment for foods. ARCH OTOLARYNGOL 1969;90:113-120.

Lee CH. A new test for the detection of food allergies and pollen and mould incompatibilities. TRANS SOC OPHTHALMOL OTOLARYNGOL 1962;3:1.

Lee CH, Williams RI, Binkley EI, Jr. Provocative inhalant testing and treatment. ARCH OTOLARYNGOL 1960;90:81.

Miller JB, A double-blind study of food extract injection therapy: a preliminary report. ANN ALLERGY 1977:39: 185-191.

Miller JB: Intradermal provocative-neutralizing food testing and subcutaneous food extract injection therapy, in OOD ALLERGY AND INTOLERANCE, Brostoff J and Challacombe SJ (Ed.). London: Bailliere Tindall, 1987, pp 932-946.

Miller JB: FOOD ALLERGY: PROVOCATIVE TESTING AND INJECTION THERAPY, Springfield, IL, Charles C Thomas, 1972

Miller JB: RELIEF AT LAST! NEUTRALIZATION FOR FOOD ALLERGY AND OTHER ILLNESSES, Charles C Thomas, 1987

Miller JB: Management of migraine headaches, in CURRENT THERAPY OF ALLERGY, Frazier CA (Ed.), New York: Medical Examination Publishing Company, Inc., 1978, pp 307-320

Miller JB: Hidden food ingredients, chemical food additives, and incomplete food labels, ANN ALLERGY, Vol. 41, No. 2, August, 1978, pp 93-98.

Miller JB: Management of food allergy, in FOOD ALLERGY: NEW PERSPECTIVES, Gerrard JW (Ed.), Charles C Thomas, Inc., September 1980.

Miller JB: The optimal-dose method of food allergy management, in OTOLARYNGOLOGIC ALLERGY, King HC (Ed.), Symposia Specialists, Inc., 1981, pp 253-283.

Miller JB: Rapid relief of varicella and infectious mononucleosis through immunotherapy, ANN ALLERGY, Vol. 47, No. 5, 1981, pp 135-136.

Miller JB: Neutralization therapy update, in ALLERGY-IMMUNOLOGIC AND MANAGEMENT CONSIDERATIONS, Spencer JT (Ed.), MEDED Publishers, Inc., 1982

For further proof, the P-N technique has even been performed and filmed double blind in animals, horses with heaves (comparable to human asthma):
Rogers SA: Provocation-Neutralization of Cough and Wheezing in a Horse, CLINICAL ECOLOGY, 5, 4, 185-187, 1987/1988.

Boris M, Schiff M, Weindorf S, et al. Bronchoprovocation blocked by neutralizing therapy, abstracted. J ALLERGY CLIN IMMUNOL 1983;71:92.

Monro J.Food allergy in migraine. PROC NUTR,1983;42:241.

Morris DL. Use of sublingual antigen in diagnosis and treatment of food allergy. ANN ALLERGY 1969;27:289-94.

O'Shea JA, et al. Double-blind study of children with hyperkinetic syndrome treated with multi-allergen disabilities. J LEARNING DISABIL 1981;14(4):189-92.

Rapp DJ. Chronic headache due to foods and air pollution. ANN ALLERGY 1978;40:289.

Rapp DJ. Hyperactivity and food allergy: are they related? ANN ALLERGY 1978;40:297.

Rapp DJ. Herpes progenitalis responding to influenza vaccine. ANN ALLERGY 1978;40:302.

Rapp DJ. Food allergy treatment for hyperkinesis. J OF LEARNING DISABILITIES 1979;12(9):42-50.

Rapp DJ. Weeping eyes in wheat allergy. Trans Am Soc Opthalmol. OTO ALLERGY 1978;18:149-50.

Rapp DJ. Double-blind confirmation and treatment of milk sensitivity. MED J AUST 1978;1:571-2.

Rea WJ, Podell RN, Williams M, Fenyves I, Sprague DE, Johnson AR. Elimination of oral food challenge reaction by injection of food extracts. ARCH OTOLARYNGOL 1984;110:248-252.

Rogers SA. Diagnosing the tight-building syndrome. ENVIR HEALTH PERSPECTIVES 1987;76:195-8.

Rogers SA. A practical approach to the person with suspected indoor air quality problems, INTERNAT CLIN NUTR REV 11:3, 126-130, July, 1991.

Rogers SA. Diagnosing the tight building syndrome or diagnosing chemical hypersensitivity. ENVIRONMENT INTERNATIONAL 1989;15:75-79.

Rogers SA. Diagnosing chemical hypersensitivity: case examples. CLIN ECOLOGY 1990;4(VI):129-34.

CRITIQUES OF NEGATIVE STUDIES ATTEMPTING TO DISCREDIT P-N

Finn R, Battcock TM. A critical study of ecology. THE PRACTITIONER 1985;229:883-5.

Forman R. A critique of evaluative studies of sublingual and intracutaneous provocative tests for food allergy. MEDICAL HYPOTHESIS 1981;7:1019-27.

Podell R. A critical review of intracutaneous and sublingual provocation and neutralization. ARCH CLIN ECOLOGY 1983;2:13-20.

Rapp DJ. Critique of the literature concerning sublingual provocation and neutralization; FOOD ALLERGY AND INTOLERANCE. Ed. Brostoff J, Challacombe SJ, Bailliere Tyndale, London, 1987:964-65.

CHEMICAL SENSITIVITY

Major awareness of chemical sensitivity was born when people developed bizarre symptoms overnight after having installed urea foam formaldehyde insulation in their homes in the 1970's. Those cases made it easy to identify cause and effect, but still because the symptoms were so diverse and unusual and contradicted the current medical paradigm, much controversy arose.

Subsequently studies showed that these levels of chemical (xenobiotics) were not that different from many ambient levels in standard homes and offices. But for the victims unlucky enough to have insidious symptoms (either from low level chronic exposure and individual genetic and biochemical susceptibility), as is often the case when medicine is stumped, psychiatric diagnoses were made.

Now, however, there is voluminous data to explain the mechanism of chemical sensitivity and the major obstacle that remains is physician education.

Because volumes of books and thousands of papers have been written on the subject of chemical sensitivity, only a small example will be provided.

Organic Solvents

Organic solvents are used in paints, fuels, adhesives, pesticides, glues, cosmetics and in the manufacture of numerous products. Millions of workers experience chronic low level exposures throughout their working lives. Consumers using the various products containing solvents sustain occasional exposures even when properly used. Accidental overexposure also occurs. In addition, the entire populace is exposed to organic solvents which find their way into our

69

air, water and food.

Recently, Wallace analyzed breath samples from 350 New Jersey residents and found benzene, perchloroethylene and trichlorethylene in 89%, 93% and 29% of the samples, respectively. Numerous other organic solvents were also detected. The long range effects of low levels of these potential carcinogens in the New Jersey residents is not known. However, low level solvent exposure can be a contributing factor to the rising cancer rate in the United States and is definitely a contributing factor to chemical sensitivity:

Wallace L, Pellizzari E, Hartwell T, et al, Concentrations of 20 volatile organic compounds in air and drinking water of 350 residents of New Jersey compared with concentrations in their exhaled breath, J OCCUP MED, 28:603-608, 1986.

Solvent exposure can cause significant depression of the central nervous system. Trichloroethylene, for example, was once used as an anesthetic gas. Often the symptoms of CNS depression occurring on either a short-term high level or chronic low level basis result in nonspecific vague symptoms from the patient. Feldman identified seven neurobehavioral problems recorded in the literature from chronic solvent exposure:

1. Memory Loss
2. Decreased Problem-Solving
3. Decreased Attention
4. Impaired Dexterity and Hand-Eye Coordination
5. Altered Reaction Time
6. Reduced Psychomotor Functions
7. Altered Personality or Mood

Indeed, organic solvents are known to cause cancer, and

chlorinated aliphatic hydrocarbon solvents are known to be hepatotoxic. It has been known for over a hundred years that chloroform damages the liver. Stimulation of liver enzymes by some solvents can cause adverse responses to ethanol and other drugs. As well, occupational and home exposure to solvents can alter immune system responses and cause lymphocytosis. A brief exposure to a mixture of solvents was shown to suppress lymphocyte function among workers.

As well, halogenated alkanes (trichloroethylene, fluorocarbons, 1,1,1,-trichloroethane, perchloroethylene and others) cause cardiac arrhythmias and sudden death by altering cardiac sensitivity to endogenous catecholamines. Sudden death has been reported from inhaling typewriter correction fluid containing 1,1,1,-trichloroethane. Likewise, kidney disease such as glomerulonephritis, or acute tubular necrosis after diesel oil exposure and Fanconi's syndrome (renal tubular acidosis) after glue sniffing have been reported.

Death occurs from cardiac sensitization with ventricular arrhythmia and respiratory depression. Acute, chronic, and even irreversible encephalopathy has been seen with glue sniffing (toluene). Most laboratories do not have the means to measure these compounds or their metabolites in patients, so that the widespread nature of solvent toxicity is not recognized.

Common sources of solvent exposure include dry cleaning fluids which many business people wear every day and are exposed to in carpets and floor cleansers as well. **EPA studies show that wearing a freshly dry-cleaned suit can give measurable levels of TCE**, for example. Dry cleaning fluids out gas the following chemicals which can be measured in the blood stream of the person working in a room

71

with a carpet that has been recently cleaned, or wearing recently dry cleaned clothes: tetrachlorethylene; trichlorethylene; 1,1,1,- trichloroethane; ethylene dichloride, mineral spirits.

EPA Project Summary, The Total Exposure Assessment Methodology (TEAM) study, Wallace LA, Office of Acid Deposition, Environmental Monitoring and Quality Assurance, Wash DC, 20460, EPA/600/s6-87/002, pp 1-14, Sept 1987.

Likewise, paints out gas toluene, xylenes, acetone, methyl ethyl ketone, methyl isobutyl ketone, and mineral spirits. And gasoline fumes can out gas benzene, toluene, xylenes, ethylene dibromide, ethylene dichloride and many other chemicals. Furthermore, common household cleansers, adhesives for furniture, and carpet backings out gas toluene, xylenes, methyl ethyl ketone, methyl isobutyl ketone, 1,1,1,-trichloroethylene, p-Dichlorobenzene and much more. And some of these such as benzene and vinyl chloride, which out gas from plastics are also known carcinogens.

There are a number of ways that these can be assayed. For example, benzene can be measured as total phenol (its main metabolite) in the urine. Styrene from plastics can be measured as mandelic acid in urine or phenylglyoxylic acid in urine. Toluene from household and office paints can be measured as hippuric acid in urine and toluene in venous blood.

Davis DL, Magee BH, Cancer and industrial chemical production, SCIENCE, 206, 1356-1358, 1978.

Feldman RG, Ricks NL, Baker EL, Neuropsychological effects of industrial toxins: a review, AMERICAN JOURNAL OF INDUSTRIAL MEDICINE, 1:211-227, 1980.

National Toxicology Program 1982, THIRD ANNUAL REPORT ON CARCINOGENS, Washington DC, Dept. of Health and Human Services.

Orris L, Tesser M. Dermatosis due to water, soaps and solvents. In H. Maibach and G. Gellin (ed). OCCUPATIONAL AND INDUSTRIAL DERMATOLOGY. Year Book Medical Publishers, 1982.

Zimmerman H, Environmental Hepatotoxicity, In HEPATOTOXICITY, Section III, pp. 279-345, Appleton-Century-Crofts/New York, 1978.

Parke DV, Activation mechanisms to chemical toxicity, ARCH TOXICOL 60: 5-15, 1987

Denkhaus W, Steldern DV, Botzenhardt U, et al, Lymphocyte subpopulations in solvent-exposed workers, INTERNATIONAL ARCHIVES OCCUPATIONAL AND ENVIRONMENTAL HEALTH, 57:109-115, 1986.

Reinhardt C, et al. Epinephrine-induced cardiac arrhythmia potential of some common industrial solvents, JOURNAL OF OCCUPATIONAL MEDICINE, 15:953-55, 1973.

Magos L, The effects of industrial chemicals on the heart. pp. 206-207. T. Balazs (ed), CARDIAC TOXICOLOGY, CRC Press 1981.

King GS, Sudden death in adolescents resulting from the inhalation of typewriter correction fluid, JOURNAL OF AMERICAN MEDICAL ASSOCIATION, 253:1604-1606, 1985.

Ravenskov U, Forseberg B, Skerfving S, Glomerulonephritis in exposure to organic solvents, ACTA MEDI SCAND.

205:575-579, 1979.

Lau SS, Marks TJ. The contribution of bromobenzene to our current understanding of chemically-induced toxicities, LIFE SCIENCES, 42: 1259-1269, 1988

Emmerson B, Toxic Nephropathy, In Wyngarden and Smith (ed), TEXTBOOK OF MEDICINE. 17th Edition, pp. 603-604, W.B. Saunders Co., 1985.

Anderson HR, et al. Epidemiology: deaths from abuse of volatile substances: a national epidemiological study, BRITISH MEDICAL JOURNAL 290:304-307, 1985.

Garriott J, et al. Death from inhalant abuse: toxicology and pathological evaluation of thirty-four cases, CLINICAL TOXICOLOGY 16:305-315, 1980.

Voigts A, Acidosis and other metabolic abnormalities associated with paint sniffing, SOUTHERN MEDICAL JOURNAL. 76:443-448, 1983.

Lazar RB, et al. Multifocal nervous system damage caused by toluene abuse, NEUROLOGY 33:1337, 1983.

The American Conference of Governmental Industrial Hygienists. THE BIOLOGICAL EXPOSURE INDICES. DOCUMENTATION OF THE THRESHOLD LIMIT VALUES, 1984. Fourth Edition, Cincinnati, OH.

Perchloroethylene

Perchloroethylene, also known as tetrachloroethylene or "perc" or PCE, is a chlorinated hydrocarbon solvent and it is commonly used in the dry cleaning industry and in metal degreasing and in the treatment of worms. So people who work in factories and people who wear dry cleaned clothes often are exposed to this as well as people working in places with carpets cleaned using these solvents. Chronic low-level exposure is known to cause impairment of brain function and decreased memory as well as potentiate cancers, malaise, dizziness, headache, increased perspiration, fatigue, incoordination, and impaired mental acuity.

Axelson O, et al, Current Aspects of Solvent Related Disorders, in DEVELOPMENTS IN OCCUPATIONAL MEDICINE, Ed. Carl Zenz, Yearbook Medical Publishers Inc., Chicago, pp. 237-59, 1977.

Sittig M, HANDBOOK OF TOXIC AND HAZARDOUS CHEMICALS, Noyes Publications, 1981.

Mutti A, et al, Nephropathies and exposure to perchloroethylene in dry-cleaners. LANCET 339: 1131-1134, 1992.

Toluene

Toluene is also known as methylbenzene, and is an aromatic hydrocarbon solvent. It is widely used in industry and of course is used in the manufacture of benzene which is used in the production of detergents, fuels, pharmaceuticals, dyes, paints, textiles (which we wear and put on furniture and walls), plastics and many other substances. Again, low-level chronic exposure can cause central nervous system depression, decreased memory, headache, dizziness, fatigue, muscular weakness, drowsiness, incoordination with staggering gait (ataxia), skin paresthesia and much more.

Toluene commonly out gasses from some plastics, paints, adhesives used for furnishings, carpeting and much more. Toluene can be measured in the blood or as hippuric acid in the urine and many prescription medications interfere with the metabolism of toluene and vice versa. When the body is not able to properly metabolize all the toluene which it is exposed to in a day, it becomes stored in the fat and is slowly released from the fat when the body is able.

Axelson O, et al, Current Aspects of Solvent Related Disorders. In DEVELOPMENTS IN OCCUPATIONAL MEDICINE (Ed. Carl Zenz), Yearbook Medical Publishers Inc., Chicago, pp. 237-59, 1977.

U.S. Environmental Protection Agency, TOLUENE, Health and Environment Effects Profile No. 160, Washington, D.C., Office of Solid Waste (April 30, 1980).

Dossing M, et al, Effect of ethanol, cimetidine, and propanol on toluene metabolism in man, INT ARCH OCCUP ENVIRON HEALTH 54:309-315 (1984).

Carlsson A, Ljungquist E, Exposure to toluene: Concentration in subcutaneous adipose tissue, SCAND J WORK ENVIRON HEALTH 8:56- 62 (1982).

Angerer J, Occupational chronic exposure to organic solvents: VII Metabolism of toluene in man, INT ARCH. OCCUP ENVIRON HEALTH 43:63-67 (1979).

Trichloroethylene

Trichloroethylene or TCE is a chlorinated hydrocarbon solvent which has a very widespread use as a metal degreaser and solvent. Alcohol may heighten the symptoms of TCE overexposure as it can with any chemical since they often compete for common pathways for detoxification and indeed TCE addiction can occur. TCE can cause peripheral neuropathy with chronic low-level exposure as well as decreased memory and impairment of the central nervous system, and cancers.

THE BRAIN AS TARGET ORGAN

TCE, as with others chemicals, is stored in the fat when the body is unable to detoxify it, when, for example there are nutrient deficiencies in the detox pathway. For example, a deficiency of zinc in the enzyme alcohol dehydrogenase will impair the ability of the body to detoxify it. Furthermore, when the body is not able to fully detoxify trichloroethylene, the brain funnels it into a different chemical pathway where it manufactures chlorol hydrate; more commonly known as "Mickey Finn" or **"knock-out drops"**. This is often responsible for the **"brain fog"** or **toxic encephalopathy** or inability to concentrate so common in people with chemical sensitivity and you can see why this symptom would wax and wane and come and go depending upon exposure to chemical, the ambient level of chemical, other chemicals in the air and drugs in the body competing with for metabolism, as well as other chemicals in the diet and the nutrient status of the body.

Because most of the indoor and outdoor air chemcials are solvents by nature, they penetrate lipids very well. The cell membrane, of course, is a lipid bilayer or "sandwich" of specialized fats or lipids and is most vulnerable to these chemicals, hence the wide variety of symptoms. But the brain is the most highly lipid organ of the body and one of the chief organs affected by chemcials. This presents a problem for physicians who are drug-oriented versus cause-oriented. For when they are presented with undiagnosable or untreatable psychiatric symptoms, they, as with other symptoms, think the only way out is to drug or cover up the symptom with medications. This only serves to further burden an already over-burdened or compromised brain and does not allow it to function better, as now it has additional chemicals to detoxify.

Cherry NM, Labreche FP, McDonald JC, Organic brain damage and occupational solvent exposure. 49:11,776-781, NOV 1992.

Sittig M, HANDBOOK OF TOXIC AND HAZARDOUS CHEMICALS, Noyes Publications, 1981.
Axelson O, et al, Current Aspects of Solvent Related Disorders. DEVELOPMENTS IN OCCUPATIONAL MEDICINE. (ed. Carl Zenz), Yearbook Medical Publishers Inc., Chicago, pp. 237-59, 1977.

Apfeldorf R, Infante P, Review of epidemiologic study results of vinyl chloride related compounds, ENVIRON HEALTH PERSPECT. 41:221-26, 1981.

Vesterberg O, Astrand I, Exposure to trichloroethylene monitored by analysis of metabolites in blood and urine, J. OCCUPATIONAL MEDICINE 18:224-226, 1976.

Ertle T, Henschler D, Muller G, Spassovski M, Metabolism of trichloroethylene in man, ARCH TOXICOL 29:171-188, 1972.

Fernandez JG, Droz PO, Humbert BE, Caperos JR, Trichloroethylene exposure: simulation of uptake, excretion and metabolism using a mathematical model, BR J INDUST MED 34:43-55, 1977.

Monster AC, Boersma G, Duba WC, Kinetics of trichloroethylene in repeated exposure to volunteers, INT ARCH OCCUP ENVIRON HEALTH 42:282-292, 1979.

Muller G, Spassovski M, Henschler D, Metabolism of trichloroethylene in man, ARCH TOXICOL 32:283-295, 1974.

Formaldehyde

Nearly every layman knows that formaldehyde sensitivity is one of the earliest examples of chemcial sensitivity. Hundreds of papers document symptoms, many of which again could masquerade as anything. In addition the literature shows us it permeats our homes, offices and outdoor environments.

And as shown earlier, the determining factor of whether or not formaldehyde creates symptoms in an individual is how replete the detoxification pathways are with nutrients.

Organophosphate Pesticides

And , as shown earlier, pesticides can cause any of the symptoms that all these other everyday chemicals can. The problem is that pesticides are virtually mixed with these chemicals we have just described so they can be sprayed. In other words, one or more of the just discussed chemicals is usually mixed with a pesticide in order to dilute it and serve as a carrier or vehicle for ease of spraying. Oddly enough, this vehicle is labelled "inert ingredients", since it is the pesticide that is the focus of attention. However, these, as you can see, are far from inert or harmless. In fact sometimes the "inert vehicle" is more damaging than the pesticide itself. In other cases, The "inert ingredient" can increase the toxicity or potentiate the pesticide by tying up precious detox enzymes.

Organophosphate pesticides are powerful inhibitors of cholinesterase, the enzyme responsible for the metabolism of acetylcholine. Acetylcholine is the neurotransmitter at parasympathetic and myoneural junctions, in autonomic ganglia, and in the brain. Poisoning occurs when the inhibition of cholinesterase leads to the accumulation of acetylcholine at the nerve synapses resulting initially in over-stimulation and then paralysis of neural transmission. This is why, for example, a bug dying of pesticide poisoning becomes very twitchy at first before he rolls over on his back and dies.

Organophosphate pesticides are classified as the safest and most widely used class of pesticides. So let's look at some facts regarding the safest ones to which the average person is exposed everyday in numerous routes (air, food, and water), for they, too can mimic any symptom.

Symptoms from organochloride pesticides can be difficult to diagnose and separate from many other illnesses and can be nebulous such as chest tightness, headache, weakness, sweating, nausea, vomiting, abdominal pain, asthma, muscle twitching, anxiety, fatigue, irritability, memory loss, restlessness, confusion, staggering, bradycardia, hypotension, depression, mood swings, and much more. And unfortunately. pesticides are ubiquitous chemicals that are found as commonly as the others above. They, too are stored in the body when the body is not able to properly detoxify them. And they can leak out of storage slowly causing chronic low-level, undiagnosable symptoms when the body gets ready to metabolize them.

References

Acheson ED, Gardner MJ, Pannet B, et al. Formaldehyde in the British Chemical Industry. LANCET. I:611. 1984

Ashford NA, Miller CA, CHEMICAL EXPOSURES, LOW LEVEL HIGH STAKES, Van Nostrand Reinhold, NY, 1991.

Battelle Columbus Laboratory. A CHRONIC INHALA-TION STUDY IN RATS AND MICE EXPOSED TO FORM-ALDEHYDE: FINAL REPORT FOR THE CHEMICAL IN-DUSTRY INSTITUTE OF TOXICOL, VOLS. 1-4, CIIT Dock-et No. 10922. Raleigh: Chemical Industry Institute of Tox-icology, 1981.

Beall JR, Ulsamer AG. Formaldehyde and Hepatotoxicity: A Review. J TOXICOL ENVIRON HEALTH, 13:1, 1984.

Beebe G, TOXIC CARPET III, P.O. Box 399086, Cincinnati, OH 45239, 1991. This book contains the 4-PC (phenylcyclohexane) story, the chemical that caused 126 out of 2000 EPA workers to become ill when a new carpet was installed in the EPA Washington mall offices.

Bernstein RS, Stayner LT, Elliott LJ, et al. Inhalation Expo-sure to formaldehyde: An Overview of its Toxicology, Epidemiology, Monitoring and Control. AMERICAN IN-DUSTRIAL HYGIENE ASSOCIATION JOURNAL, 45:778, 1984.

Bernstein RS, Falk H, Turner DR, Melius JM. Nonoccupational Exposures to Indoor Air Pollutants: A Survey of State Programs and Practicies. AMER J PUB HEALTH, 74:1020, 1984.

Blair A, Stewart P, O'berg M, et al. Mortality Among Industrial Workers Exposed to Formaldehyde. J NAT CAN-CER INSTIT. 76:1071, 1984.

Breysse P. The Immediate and Long-Term Effects of Form-aldehyde. COMMENTS ON TOXICOLOGY. June, 1988.

Broder I, Corey P, Cole P, et al. Comparison of Health of Occupants and Characteristics of Houses Among Control

Homes and Homes Insulated with Urea Formaldehyde Foam. II. Initial Health and House Variables and Exposure-Response Relationships.ENVIRONMENTAL RESEARCH. 45:156, 1988.

Broder I, Corey P, Cole P, et al. Comparison of Health of Occupants and Characteristics of Houses Among Control Homes and Homes Insulated with Urea Formaldehyde Foam. II. Health and House Variables Following Remedial Work. ENVIRONMENTAL RESEARCH. 45:179, 1988.
Broughton A, Thrasher JD. Antibodies and altered cell mediated immunity in formaldehyde exposed humans COMMENTS ON TOXICOLOGY, 2:155, 1988.

Casanovea M, Heck Hd'A. Further Studies of the Metabolic Incorporation and Covalent Binding of Inhaled [3H]-and [14C] Formaldehyde in Fischer-334 Rats: Effects of Glutathione Depletion. TOXICOL APP PHARMACOL, 89:105, 1987.

Dally KA, Hanrahan LP, Woodbury MA. Formaldehyde Exposure in Nonoccupational Environments. ARCH ENVIRON HEALTH, 36:277, 1981.

Environmental Protection Agency. FORMALDEHYDE HEALTH RISK ASSESSMENT. U.S. Environmental Protection Agency, Washington, DC, 1987.

French D, Edsall JT. The Reactions of Formaldehyde with Amino Acids and Proteins. ADVANCES IN PROTEIN CHEMISTRY, 2:278, 1945.

Gamble J. Effects of Formaldehyde on the Respiratory System. In: FORMALDEHYDE TOXICITY (Gibson JE, ED.) New York: Hemisphere Publishing Company, p. 175, 1983.

Gosslin RE, Smith RP, Hodge HC. CLINICAL TOXICOLO-
GY OF COMMERCIAL PRODUCTS, 5th Edition. Baltimore: Williams and Wilkins, 1984.

Gupta K. HEALTH EFFECTS OF FORMALDEHYDE. US
Consumer Product Safety Commission, Washington DC,
1984.

Gupta K, Ulsamer AG, Preuss PW. Formaldehyde in Indoor
Air: Sources and Toxicity. ENVIRONMENT INTERNA-
TIONAL, 8:38, 1982.

Gupta KC, Ulsamer AG, Preuss PW. Formaldehyde in Indoor
Air: Sources and Toxicity. ENVIRONMENT INTERNA-
TIONAL. 8:349, 1982.

Hayes WJ, PESTICIDES STUDIED IN MAN, ORGANIC
PHOSPHOROUS PESTICIDES, 284-435, Williams and
Wilkins, Baltimore, 1982.

Horvath EP, Anderson H, Pierce WE, et al. Effects of
Formaldehyde on the Mucous Membranes and Lungs. J
AMER MED ASSOC. 259:701, 1988.

Kilburn KH, Warshaw R, Thronton JC. Formaldehyde
Impairs Memory, Equilibrium and Dexterity in Histology
Technicians: Effects which Persist for Days After Eposure.
ARCH ENVIRON HEALTH, 42:17, 1987.

Kilburn KH, Warshaw R, Thronton JC. Formaldehyde
Impairs Memory, Equilibrium and Dexterity in Histology
Technicians: Effects which Persist for Days After Eposure.
ARCH ENVIRON HEALTH, 42:117, 1987.

Konopinski VJ. Seasonal Formaldehyde Concentrations in
an office Building. AMER INDUST HYGIENE ASSOC,

146:65, 1985.

LaMarte FP, Merchant JH, Casale TB. Acute Systemic Reactions To Carbonless Copy Paper Associated with Histamine Release. J AMER MED ASSOC, 260:248, 1988.

Mago L, The Effects of Industrial Chemicals on the Heart, 206-207 in Balazo T, ed., CARDIAC TOXICOLOGY, CRC PRESS, Boca Raton, FL 1981.
Marks JG, Trautlein JJ, Zwillich W, Demers LM. Contact Urticaria and Airway Obstruction from Carbonless Copy Paper. J AMER MED ASSOC, 252:1038, 1984.

Morgan KT, Patterson DL, Gross EA. Formaldehyde and the Nasal Mucociliary Apparatus. In: FORMALDEHYDE: TOXICOLOGY, EPIDEMIOLOGY, MECHANISMS. New York: Marcel Dekker, Inc., p. 193, 1983.

National Academyof Science, Report of the Federal Panel on Formaldehyde. ENVIRONMENTAL HEALTH PERSPECTIVES, 43:139, 1982.

Olsen JH, Dossing M. Formaldehyde Induced Symptoms in Day Care Centers. AMERICAN INDUSTRIAL HYGIENE ASSOCIATION JOURNAL, 43:366, 1982.

Rea WJ, CHEMICAL SENSITIVITY, VOL.I., Lewis Publ., Boca Raton, 1992.

Rea WJ, CHEMICAL SENSITIVITY, VOL.II., Lewis publ., Boca Raton, 1992.

Ritchie IM, Lehnen RG. Formaldehyde-related Health Complaints of Residents Living in Mobile and Conventional Homes. AMER PUB HEALTH. 77:323, 1987.

Rogers SA, Chemical Sensitivity: Breaking the Paralyzing Paradigm, Parts I in INTERN MED WORLD REP., 7:3, 1, 15-17 Feb 1 1992, Part II ibid 7:6, 2, 21-31, Mar 1, 1992, Part III ibid 7:8, 13-16, 32-33, 40-41, Apr 15, 1992.

Samet JM, Marbury MC, Spengler JD. Respiratory Effects of Indoor Air Pollution. J ALLER CLIN IMMUNOL, 79:685, 1987.

Scott CS, Margosches EH. Cancer Epidemiology Relevant to Formaldehyde. J ENVIRON SCI HEALTH, Part C. 3:107, 1985.

Shusterman DJ, Blanc PC, OCCUPATIONAL MEDICINE: STATE OF THE ART REVIEWS. UNUSUAL OCCUPATIONAL DISEASES. 7:3, Jul-Sept 1992, Hanley and Belfus Inc, Philadelphia.

Sterling DA. Volatile Organic Compounds in Indoor Air: An Overview of Sources, Concentrations and Health Effects. IN: INDOOR AIR AND HUMAN HEALTH (Gammage RB, Kaye SV, Jacobs VA, Eds. Chelsea:Lewis Publishers, Inc., Boca Raton Fl, p.387, 1985.

Stock TH, Mendez SR. A Survey of Typical Exposures to Formaldehyde in the Houston Area. AMERICAN INDUSTRIAL HYGIENE ASSOCIATION JOURNAL, 46:313, 1985.

Swenberg JA, Gross EA, Randall HW, Barrow BS. The Effect of Formaldehyde on Cytotoxicity and Cell Proliferation, ibid, p 225.

Thrasher J, Broughton A, THE POISONING OF OUR HOMES AND WORKPLACES, Antigen Assay Labs, 1-800-522-2611, 1984.

Thrasher JD, Madison R, Broughton A, Gard Z. Building-Related Illness and Antibodies to Conjugates of Formaldehyde, Toluene Diisocyanate and Trimellitic Anhydride. AMER INDUST MED, 15:187, 1989.

Thrasher JD, Wojdani A, Cheung G, Heuser G. Evidence for Formaldehyde Antibodies and Altered Cellular Immunity in Subjects Exposed to Formaldehyde in Mobile Homes. ARCH ENVIRON HEALTH, 42:347, 1987.

Thrasher JD, Broughton A, Micevich P. Antibodies and Immune Profiles of Individuals Occupationally Exposed to Formaldehyde: Six Case Reports. AMER J INDUSTR MED, 14:479, 1988.

Ulsamer AG, Beall JR, Kang HK, Frazier JA. Overview of Health Effects of Formaldehyde. In: HAZARD ASSESSMENT OF CHEMICALS: CURRENT DEVELOPMENTS. New York: Academic Press, Inc., Vol. 3, p. 338, 1984.

Wallace L, Pelliazzari E, Harwell T, et al. Concentrations of 20 Volatile Organic Compounds in Air and Drinking Water of 350 Residents of New Jersey Compared with Concentrations in Their Exhaled Breath. J OCCUP MED, 38:603, 1986.

Wilhelmsson B, Homlstrom M. Positive Formaldehyde Test after Prolonged Formaldehyde Exposure by Inhalation. LANCET, 2(8551):164, 1987.

Woodbury MA, Zenz C. Formaldehyde in the Home Environment: Prenatal and Infant Exposures. In: FORMALDEHYDE TOXICITY (Gibson JE, Ed.) New York: Hemisphere Publishing Corporation, p.203, 1983.

Zimmerman N. The Carcinogenic Potential of Formaldehyde. COMMENTS ON TOXICOLOGY. June, 1988.

It is a quantum leap for many to master the chemistry in order to be able to comprehend the paradigm shift in medicine that chemical sensitivities ushers in. But once this knowledge is conquered, you can begin to appreciate what others have observed for over two decades: that **anyone can react to any chemical with any organ as the target organ at any time.**

And indeed, chemical sensitivity can trigger diseases of the skin, lung, musculoskeletal system, gastrointestinal, hepatic, renal, cardiac, endocrine and nervous systems. No medical conditions or symptoms are exempt.

XENOBIOTICS MIMIC ANY DISEASE

Many foreign chemicals can get into the system and damage enzymes and regulatory proteins, thereby creating difficult-to-diagnose symptoms. And they can mimic any symptom or disease. And this is understandable since behind every diagnostic and therapeutic dilemma is a cause. Heavy metals, for example, are common. Lead poisoning in children is a common cause of failure to mature mentally. Likewise, years of aluminum-containing antacids can accumulate aluminum in the brain and potentiate neurofibrillary tangles coincident with Alzheimer's disease.

Likewise, mercury (used in dental amalgams and non-prescription medicines and in fungicides) can mimic psychiatric symptoms.

Ngim CH, FOO SC, Boey KW, Teyaratnam J, Chronic neurological effects of elemental mercury in dentists. BRIT J INDUSTR MED, 49:11, 782-790, 1992.

Pesticides are among the most damaging and ubiquitous chemicals in the normal environment. They are not only used in homes, offices, on lawns, but in plastics, foods, and other areas. Pesticides, herbicides, fungicides, rodenticides, etc. are all formulated with one thing in mind: to kill life. United States government's EPA pesticide manual shows that any symptom is possible.Likewise, people with chemical sensitivity who do not have the ability to detoxify inhaled chemicals as rapidly as the average person, tend to store these chemicals.

Volatile organic compounds, such as xylene, benzene, toluene, formaldehyde and more, can mimic any disease and a host of symptoms that are undiagnosable. The primary target organs are the brain and peripheral nervous system, the respiratory system, and the gastrointestinal system. But no part of the body is immune. In fact the immune system itself is quite vulnerable to damage from pesticides.

The United States government's Environmental Protection Agency has published an excellent book, "Recognition and Management of Pesticide Poisonings" (United States Environmental Protection Agency, EPA-540/9-80-005, January, 1982, Third Edition).

In it they remind us that,"**rarely are particular manifestations always present in poisonings by a given chemical and many poisonings are characterized by unexpected symptoms. Furthermore there are usually many causes of particular signs and symptoms.**" And the EPA goes on to explain that "Not all manifestations of illness are included. **Some symptoms,** such as dizziness and weakness are caused by so many chemicals by either direct or indirect mechanisms that they **have little value diagnostically.**" In other words, the symptom label is useless. It is the underlying cause, such as pesticide poisoning that has medical significance.

Furthermore the United States Environmental Protection Agency through Gitendra Saxena (Ed) produced a book "Hazardous Assessment of Chemicals", Vol 6 (Hemisphere Publishing Corp., 1989).

In there they show a multitude of references and state that immuno- suppressive actions have been demonstrated for many pesticides, and that the data illustrates a wide range of sensitivity to immuno-suppression leading to increased susceptibility to infection, decreased cell mediated immunity, depressed T-cell lymphocyte function, depressed levels of serum complement, altered responses to T and B cell mitogenes, decreased spleen and thymus weight and altered natural killer cell cytotoxicity.

For example, "Altered susceptibility to infection following the exposure to pesticides provides another measure of chronic immuno-toxicity." In other words pesticide exposures can not only mimic many diseases, but create many undiagnosable problems (like recurrent infections) that will go on to actually become known "labels" or diseases or syndromes or conditions.

In case there is the slightest misconception left, let me put it another way: **No matter how "incredible" or "untreatable" or "hopeless" a condition may be, there has not been a proper medical investigation until chemical triggers have been ruled out.** These 2 books by the U.S. government EPA show us how pesticides, as one example, can mimic nearly any disease since they can cause a wide range of symptoms in humans.

As another example, take something as seemingly "closed" as Parkinson's disease, which most neurologists will treat with drugs only. It is common knowledge that after a while, the drugs lose their effectiveness and the disease relentlessly progresses. But everyday chemicals, including pesticides, can alter chemical detoxification. We now know how to slow up Parkinson's progression and in some cases reverse the severity, without drugs.

Fahn S. "The Endogenous Toxin Hypothesis of the Etiology of Parkinson's Disease and a Pilot Trial of High-Dosage Antioxidants in an Attempt to Slow the Progression of the Illness, in"BIOCHEMISTRY AND HEALTH IMPLICATIONS, New York Academy Press,1989.

Calne DB, Eisen A, McGeer E. Spencer P. "Alzheimer's Disease, Parkinson's Disease, and Motoneurone Disease: Interaction between Ageing and Environment?" LANCET. Pp.1067-70, Nov. 8. 1986.

Schuster L. "Frequent Use of Herbicides May Triple the Risk of Parkinson's, FAMILY PRACTICE NEWS. P.49, Feb 15, 1993.

Steventon GB, Heafield MTE, Waring RH, et al. "Xenobiotic Metabolism in Parkinson's Disease," NEUROLOGY. Vol. 39, pp.883-87, 1989.

"Parkinson's Disease: One Illness or Many Syndromes? "(Editorial) LANCET. Vol.339, no.8804, pp.1263-64, 1992.

Steventon GB, Williams AC, Waring, RH, Pall HS. Xenobiotic Metabolism in Motoneuron Disease," LANCET. Pp 644-47, Sept.17, 1988.

Steventon, GB, Heafield MTE, Sturman S, et al. "Xenobiotic Metabolism in Alzheimer's Disease," NEUROLOGY. Vol 40, pp 1095-98, 1990.

Chapman LJ. "Parkinsonism and Industrial Chemicals," LANCET, Aug 12, 1989, pp 356-57.

Williams S. "Neglected Neurotoxicants, " SCIENCE. Vol. 248, p 958, May 25, 1990

PESTICIDES: THE GREATEST MIMIC OF ALL

Pesticides are ubiquitously and surreptitiously used in commercial businesses and can masquerade as flu-like illnesses, mental disease, neurologic disease, colds, headaches, body aches, sore throats, chemical sensitivity, asthma, chronic fatigue, and more. And there need not be the presumed reduction of RBC acetylcholinesterase activity. This blood test is too insensitive to serve as a diagnostic tool for chronic poisoning. It is only useful in a massive acute poisoning. And sometimes it is not the pesticide anyway that triggers symptoms, but the "inert" vehicle, as described.

Dogson MJ, Block GD, Parkinsons DK, Organophosphate Poisoning in Office Workers. J OCCUP MED, 28,: 434, 1986

LIST OF PESTICIDE PRODUCTS' INERT INGREDIENTS. Office of Pesticides & Toxic Substances, U.S. EPA, Jan 15, 1992

Kaloyanova FP, El Batowi MA, HUMAN TOXICOLOGY OF PESTICIDES, CRC Press, Boca Raton, FL, 1991

Arlien-Soborg, P, SOLVENT NEURO-TOXICITY, CRC Press, Boca Raton FL, 1992

Furthermore, pesticides may damage hormone receptors and mimic classic glandular disorders such as hyperthyroidism(Adler, T. Dioxins Meddle With The Thyroid Hormone. SCIENCE NEWS 144: 24, 391).

As well pesticides can trigger infertility or endometriosis (Gibbons A, Dioxin Tied to Endometriosis, SCIENCE 262: 1373, Nov 26, 1993)

Furthermore, everyday pesticides can trigger not only seizures, visual, respiratory, abdominal, neurological, metabolic, hormonal and gastrointestinal sysmptoms, but cardiac arrhythmias. And as they become mobilized from body fat stores, they can cause baffling repeated relapses.

Bardin PG , Van Eeden SF, et al, Organophosphate & Carbamate Poisoning. A Review, ARCH INTERN MED, 154: 1433-1441, July 11 1994.

This should serve as a cursory example that pesticides, heavy metals, and other everyday chemicals can mimic many symptoms for which drugs are blindly prescribed. Thus a search for them and their effects is indicated.

PROOF OF CHEMICAL SENSITIVITY

An offshoot of the serial dilution titration is the provocation-neutralization test which uses miniscule doses of xenobiotics to test for chemical sensitivity, as has been described earlier in this monograph. This technique was published in the United States Government's National Institutes of Health medical journal ENVIRONMENTAL HEALTH PERSPECTIVES and the governments' EPA "Indoor Air Referenced Bibliography" and other places.

In the office, in order to determine chemical sensitivity, it is common to test to chemicals in a single-blind fashion. In other words, the patient is given several normal saline injections or placebos before he is given the real test. Therefore, he does not know when he is being tested to the real thing and malingering can be ruled out. If the antigen has a sting or a bite to it, then single-blind testing to another antigen that stings to which he is not sensitive can be added.

Further proof for chemical sensitivity can come from measuring before exposure and after exposure blood tests, such as formic acid levels, detox enzymes such as urinary hippuric acid levels, or the accumulation of xenobiotics or their breakdown products. Before and after liver enzymes, nutrients, pulmonary functions, and even photos can often substantiate the subjective symptoms.

HEALING THE GUT CAN HALT THE VICIOUS CYCLE OF DISEASE

Intestinal Dysbiosis and Intestinal Hyperpermeability

It is well-known that the intestinal flora can be significantly altered by diet, antibiotics, hormones, and other factors. The flora itself is very important for determining the integrity of the intestinal barrier. For example,if abnormal amounts of organisms (even those that are not normally pathogenic) are present, they can inflame the intestinal lining. Likewise, undetected food allergies can also cause inflammation of the intestinal lining.

When this lining is inflamed, several things occur:

(1) Number one, large food particles that normally do not cross the intestinal barrier are allowed through intersti tial (between the cells) spaces into the bloodstream. When the body sees these "new"or foreign large parti cles that it has never seen before, it mounts a defensive attack and antibodies are formed. New food allergies can arise and also autoimmune antibodies can arise which will lead to autoimmune diseases. If similar antigenic sites exist on thyroid or joint spaces or in the lung, for example, then an autoimmune phenomenon can occur whenever a particular antigen is eaten or encountered.

(2) Likewise, a major part of the detoxification pathway of the body is in the lining of the intestine. When it becomes inflamed, a major part of the detox capability has been lost and chemical sensitivity can start.

(3) The third major problem that occurs from intestinal inflammation is that the carrier proteins which normal

94

ly attach onto minerals and carry them into the blood stream can be lost or damaged. Therefore nutrient deficiencies occur which then can lead to other symptoms and diseases.

(4) Furthermore, an inflamed or leaky gut, or hyperpermeable gut can go on to allow the absorption of toxins which can cause fatigue and body achiness and other symptoms.

Therefore, it is important to test for intestinal dysbiosis and abnormal amounts of organisms, whether they be considered pathogenic or not (such as the yeast Candida albicans). For, a hyperpermeable gut, which signifies damage to the intestinal mucosa, is important to diagnose so that it can be corrected and stop the vicious cycle of disease. For one imbalanced organism or food allergy can, as described, initiate an autoimmune disease that affects any or all organs of the body.

Sometimes correction of the intestinal flora can be quite simple, like having the proper probiotics (species of Lactobacillus acidophilus, for example) in the intestine. These possess many advantageous effects which help to improve health. Likewise the Bifidobacteria enhance immunity, lower cholesterol, suppress tumors, enhance hepatic function and decrease free phenols, for example.

As a simple example, the presence of a bacterium, Helicobacter pylori, can mimic ulcers. If this were not diagnosed, ulcer therapy like H-2 blockers and antacids could be prescribed indefinitely and these would impair the absorption of priceless minerals. This mineral loss in turn could go on to cause any number of symptoms from hypertension, chemical sensitivity, chronic fatigue or chronic low back pain to angina or sudden death. Or the pain could prompt an unnecessary and not at all currative surgery. And undiagnosed H. pylori can cause gastric cancer.

The intestines contain hundreds of bacteria and fungi. The purposes are many. Some bacteria help nourish the intestinal lining, some help us manufacture vitamins, but most help to literally rot or break down our food into smaller molecular pieces so that it is easily absorbed.

But when antibiotics are taken, as they frequently are in the U.S., they do not kill all the intestinal organisms. (It's a good thing or we would die.) Some of the organisms are resistant(like C. difficile, H pylori, C. albicans).So having had some of their competition annihilated, they grow unencumbered and multiply rapidly. And this overgrowth can inflame the gut and make it hyperpermeable.

Sometimes the overgrowth is of certain species of bacteria, protozoa, mold (or fungi or yeasts) which are particularly antibiotic-resistant. When this happens (as does in a host that is especially compromised by undetected nutrient deficiencies) these organisms are also capable of making toxins that cause hyperpermeability of the gut, leading to further food allergy, auto- immune antibodies and more. Hence we see one more mechanism where the sick must get sicker when drugs are used in place of searching for a treatable cause.

Also the host (patient) can become sick from the absorption of these toxins. Besides damaging the immune system in a myriad of ways, they can mimic many diseases. In fact, some mycotoxins (toxins produced by molds, such as afla-toxins) are known to be strong carcinogens and only extremely small amounts are needed to initiate a cancer.

96

One normally harmless yeast or mold which rallies in a compromised host (such as one not playing with a full deck of nutrients) after antibodies are given is Candida albicans. Its overgrowth in the intestine can mimic many diverse symptoms.

Needless to say, cultures of the stool can be done to identify these organisms, tests for intestinal hyperpermeability can be done, diets can be prescribed that foster the growth of healthier gastro-intestinal tracts, and products can be prescribed to decrease the growth of these abnormal amounts of organisms.

References

Alexander JG: Allergy in the gastrointestinal tract. LANCET, 2:1264, 1975.

Boren T et al. Attachment of H. pylori to human gastric epithelium mediated by blood group antigens. SCIENCE 1993; 262:1892-5.

Buist R: The Malfunctional "mucosal barrier" and food allergies. INTERNATIONAL CLIN NUTR REV 3:1-4, 1983.

Chaitow L, Trenev N, PROBIOTICS, Thorsons, London, 1990.

Doube A collins AJ: Is the gut intrinsically abnormal in rheumatoid arthritis? ANN RHEUM DIS 47: 617-19, 1988.

Fedotin MS. Helicobacter pylori and peptic ulcer disease. POSTGRAD MED 1993; 94: 38-45.

Forbes GM et al. Duodenal ulcer treated with H. pylori

eradication. LANCET 1994; 343: 543.

Iwata K: A review of the literature of drunken symptoms due to yeasts in the gastrointestinal tract, in Iwata K (ed): YEASTS AND YEAST-LIKE MICROORGANISMS IN MEDICAL SCIENCE. Tokyo, University of Tokyo Press, 1976, pp. 260-268.

James J and Warrin RP: An assessment of the role of Candida albicans and food yeasts in chronic urticaria. BR J DERM, 84:227-237, 1971.

Jenkins RT et al: Increased intestinal permeability in patients with rheumatoid arthritis: A side effect of oral NSAID therapy? BR J RHEUMATOL 26: 103-07, 1987.

Kerdelko NM, Allergy in chronic monilial vaginitis, ANN ALLER 29, 95-96, 1971.

Liebeskind A, Candida albicans as an allergic factor, ANN ALLERG 20: 394-396, 1962.

Miles MR, Olsen L, Roberts A: Recurrent vaginal candidiasis; importance of an intestinal reservoir. JAMA, 238: 1836-1837, 1977.

Mitsuoka T, Bifidobacteria and their role in human health, J INDUST. MICROBIOL 6 (1990) 263-268.

Mott GE, et al, Lowering of serum cholesterol by intestinal bacteria in cholesterol-fed piglets, LIPIDS, 8:428-431, 1973.

Nelson RD, Herron JM, McCormack RJ, et al: Two mechanisms of inhibition of human lymphocyte proliferation by soluble yeast mannan poly saccharide. INFECT IMMUN, 43: 104101046, 1984.

Odds FC: CANDIDA AND CANDIDOSIS. Baltimore, University Park Press, 1979, p.140.

Parsonnet J, H. pylori as a risk factor for gastric cancer. EURO J GASTROENT HEPAT 1993; 5(suppl 1): S103-S107.

Pearson A, et al, Intestinal permeability in children with Crohn's disease and cardiac disease BR MED J 285: 20-21, 1982.

Reinhardt M: Macromolecular absorption of food antigens in health and disease. ANN ALLERGY 53: 597, 1984.

Rex DK. An etiologic approach to management of duodenal and gastric ulcers. J FAM PRACT 1994; 38" 600-6007.

Rippon JW: MEDICAL MYCOLOGY. Second edition. Philadelphia, WBB Saunders Co, 1982, p.499.

Rosenberg EW, Below PW, Skinner RB, Crutcher N: Response to: Crohn's disease and psoriasis. NEW ENG J MED, 308:101, 1983.

Seelig MS: Mechanisms by which antibiotics increase the incidence and severity of candiasis and alter the immunological defenses. BACTERIAL REV, 30: 442-459, 1966.

Shahini KM, Friend BA, Nutritional and therapeutic aspects of Lactobacilli, J APPL NUTR, 37:2, 136-165, 1973.

Simon GL, Gorbach SL, Intestinal flora in health and disease, PHYSIOLOGY OF THE GASTROINTESTINAL TRACT, Johnson LR (ed), 1361-1380, Raven Press, NY, 1981.

Smith AW et al. Blood group antigens and H. pylori infections. LANCET 1994; 343:543

Suzuki M et al. H. pylori elicitis gastric mucosal cell damage associated with neutrophil-derived toxic oxidants. EURO J GASTROENT HEPAT 1993; 5(SUPPL 1): S35-S39.

Tamura K et al. Ammonia is produced by H. pylori, related to superoxide generation in situ, as a major factor in acute gastritis. EURO J GASTROENT HEPAT 1993; 5(suppl 1): S51-S56.

Walker W: Transmucosal pasage of antigens, in Schmidt E (Ed): FOOD ALLERGY. Raven Press, NY 1988.

Wilcox et al., Gastrointestinal hemorrage and the use of NSAIDs, ARCH INTERN MED, 154: 42, 1994.

Witkin SS: Defective immune responses in patients with recurrent Candidiasis. INFECTIONS IN MEDICINE, pp. 129-132, May/June 1985.

Witkin SS, YuIR, Ledger WJ: Inhibiton of Candida albicans-induced lymphocyte proliferation by lymphocytes and sera from women with recurrent vaginitis. AM J OBSTET GYNECOL, 147: 809-811, 1983.

INTESTINAL ORGANISMS CAN LEAK INTO THE BLOOD STREAM

It is well-known, for example, that antibiotics can cause an overgrowth of Clostridium difficile, that in turn mimics severe colitis. And Helicobactor pylor (Campylobacter pylori) infection can mimic intractable ulcers, and can go on to cause cancers. Likewise bacterial and fungal translocations have been recorded with election micrography showing abdominal organisms are capable of passing into other tissues via the blood stream causing a wide array of "undiagnosable" and "untreatable" symptoms.

Alexander JW, et al, The process of intestinal microbial translocation, ANN SURG 1990: 212 (4): 496-512

Even if the organisms do not pass from the gut into the system, much damage can occur in the intestine that in turn affects literally any part of the rest of the body (hyperpermeable gut pathology as previously described).

INTESTINAL HEALING

Fortunately there are many natural components which exert a trophic or healing effect on the gut wall. One example of the multiple materials there are available to heal the gut is L-glutamine, a simple amino acid that promotes healing of damaged intestinal mucosa. In fact it is so healing that it even protects against damage induced by radiation to the gut.

Many of these modalities, as exemplified here are very important, especially when they can even protect against radiation damage. It is a shame they are not as well known as prescription drugs which do not have anywhere near this protective and healing capability.

Klein S, Glutamine: An Essential Non-essential Amino Acid for the Gut. GASTROENTEROLOGY, 1990:99(1): 279-81

Klimberg vs, et al, Prophylactic Glutamine Protects the Intestinal Mucosa From Radiation Injury. CANCER, 1990, 1:66 (1): 62-8

Shrive E, et al Glutamine in Treatment of Peptic Ulcer, TEX J MED, 53: 840-43, 1957

BIOCHEMICAL INDIVIDUALITY,
TARGET ORGAN SPECIFICITY, AND TOTAL LOAD

One of the most difficult yet logical concepts for people unfamiliar with environmental medicine to grasp is that of biochemical individuality. We don't all just look different; we are different biochemically. Thousands of papers in the scientific literature show how only some people will develop lupus antibodies after taking certain prescription medications that are safe for the vast majority. Hydralizine and procainamide are examples of commonly prescribed drugs that can initiate or start lupus. Numerous studies have been done on the enzyme AHH (aryl hydroxyl hydratase) which makes the difference of whether or not a person will get emphysema or cancers from certain chemicals that other people are unaffected by.

Even the U.S. EPA when they installed thousands of square feet of new carpet in one of their Washington mall offices saw the uniqueness of each person and biochemical individuality. For, out of 2,000 workers, only 126 developed environmental illness or chemical sensitivity. And out of those, no two people had the exact same symptoms.

Ert V, Clayton JW, Crabbe CL, Walsh JW, Indentification and Characterization of 4-phenylcyclohexene: An Emission Product from New Carpeting. No. Ots-0288-0596 to U.S. Environmental Protection Agency, Wash DC, Jan 8, 1987, EPA.

Indoor Air Quality & Work Environmental Study: Employee Survey, Vol 1, US EPA, Wash DC, Nov, 1989

Another publication by the United States government's Environmental Protection Agency, Washington, D.C., was edited by Gitendra Saxena, entitled HASARD ASSESSMENT OF CHEMICALS, Vol 6, Hemisphere Publishing Corp., New York, 1989. In there they state "Individuals vary in their susceptibility to the toxic effect of hazardous chemicals. A number of factors including genetic predisposition, age, gender, nutritional status, pre-existing disease, and concomitant exposure to other compounds are all capable of modifying an individual's response to a toxicant. Human populations are a variable with respect to diet, occupation, and home environment, activity patterns, and other cultural factors. The following are factors that influence individual susceptibility to the toxic effect of exposure to xenobiotics:

> genetic predisposition
> age
> gender
> nutritional status
> diet
> body composition
> concomitant disease
> pre-existing pathology
> toxicant interaction
> home environment
> occupational factors
> activity patterns
> cultural factors"

So no two people have the same set of circumstances at one time. So they all are capable of reacting differently to the same exposure. And in addition, an individual may not have the same set of operant circumstances with subsequent exposures, so his reactions and symptoms can vary from one exposure to the next. This really confuses a physician unschooled in xenobiotic detoxication biochemistry and environmental medicine.

"In a recent report, the GAO (1986) defined the concept of using safety factors to place quantitative limits on exposure to environmental chemicals, specifically pesticides. The safety factor

103

was defined as a "number intended to provide a margin of safety to account for inherent uncertainty in projecting the results of animal toxicology studies to humans."

"The total safety factor for pesticides is usually ten-fold to account for the differences between humans and test animals and ten-fold for the differences in the sensitivity among different people. An experimentally derived no observable effect-level (NOEL) can then be divided by the safety factor to yield the quantitative estimate of acceptable daily intake (ADI). For pesticides, ADI is defined as "a person's daily intake of a pesticide residue which, during a lifetime, is not expected to cause an appreciable health risk on the basis of all facts known at the time (GAO, 1986)".

This translates to the fact that safety levels of pesticides are merely a mathematical guess based on information that is over a decade old. They are not based in scientific fact. Nor do they take into account the vast amount of scientific data, for example, that has been alluded to in this monograph.

Furthermore they go on to state that there is tremendous genetic variation in the ability of members of the human population to detoxify or metabolize foreign chemicals. "Human populations show considerable variation in the metabolism of many xenobiotics". This means that for an unspecified percentage (that could be quite significant), many of these chemicals are alarmingly unsafe.

There are many genetic types where the underlying genetic polymorphism has been described and the effects on human sensitivity to toxins has been investigated. Examples are given of the single recessive autosomol gene for slow phenotypes who are termed slow acetylators. These are the people that can develop a lupus-like rheumatoid syndrome when given the antihypertensive drug hydralazine or the anti-arrhythmic agent procainamide. And these people are more prone to developing cancers when exposed to environmental arylamines. There can be up to a 13-fold difference in the acetylation rate among people and several studies suggest that slow acetylators are at much greater risk for bladder cancer. And of course they are at greater risk for chemical sensitivity in general.

Debrisoquine is an old antihypertensive, whose detoxication is also regulated by the cytochrome P-450 system and has been shown to have an over 20-fold difference among people in their ability to metabolize this:

Barbeau A, Roy M Paris S, Cloutier T, Plane L, Poirer L, Ecogenetics of Parkinson's Disease: For Hydroxylation of Debrisoquine, LANCET 1213-1216, Nov 30, 1985

But remember the government has decided (1986) that we need only assume that people have a ten-fold vaiability in ability to handle dangerous pesticides.

Other drugs have over 160-fold variation in the ability of people to detoxify them. Aryl hydrocarbon hydroxylase (AAH) is an enzyme used to metabolize polycyclic aromatic hydrocarbons. If these common environmental hydrocarbons are not properly metabolized in the cytochrome P-450 system, cancer is a definite outcome with many. And again, there is an over 28-fold range in the AAH activity among people. And in fact, it has been used as a marker for cancer susceptibility. Likewise the enzyme epoxide hydrolase is extremely important in determining whether or not an environmental chemical becomes a carcinogen and researchers have demonstrated an over 8-fold variation in the liver epoxide hydrolase activity among humans.

The government-sponsored study by Saxena also goes on to show that there is tremendous variation in target tissues. In other words, for a particular chemical, one person may have damage to the brain, another the heart, and another to the kidneys. The bottom line that can be drawn from this government publication is that there is such biochemical and genetic variation among people that it is down right absurd for any institution (scientific, medical or otherwise) to proclaim something as safe for everyone at a specific level.

This brings us to the other concept that is difficult to grasp when you have a drug-oriented view of medicine, and that is target organ specificity. If hundreds of people are exposed to a pesticide, for example, most will have no symptoms. Some will have excruciating headaches, others will have nausea, others abdominal cramps, others will have disorientation, etc. The target organ for a response to a chemical or antigen can be anywhere. It depends upon the specific person, their heredity, diet, lifestyle, xenobiotic detoxification pathway, nutrients, current total body burden of xenobiotics (foreign chemicals), and much more. It's definitely a package deal.

Or if we want to look at a much simpler example, another paper shows that there is no consistent association between viable mold growth and sensitization to molds. This is because it is an individual problem, just as the EPA carpet was:

Wickman M, Graveson S, Nordwall SL, Pershogan G, Sundell J, Indoor viable dust-bound microfungi in relation to residential characteristics, living habits, and symptoms in atopic and controlled children. J ALLERGY CLIN IMMUNOL 89: 752-9, 1992.

In summary, there is a vast amount of data proving a wide biochemical individuality among people. This demonstrates the ludicrous lack of knowledge for institutions that attempt to assert otherwise.

Calabrese EJ, POLLUTIONS AND HIGH GROUPS: THE BIO-LOGICAL BASIS OF INCREASED HUMAN SUSCEPTIBILI-TY TO ENVIRONMENTAL AND OCCUPATIONAL POL-LUTANTS, J Wiley & Sons, NY 1978.

Scriver CR, Beaudet AL, Sly WS, Valle D, ed, THE METABOL-IC BASIS OF INHERITED DISEASE, VOL I & II, 6TH Ed, McGraw-Hill, NY, 1989.

Rea WJ, CHEMICAL SENSITIVITY VOL I, Lewis Publ (CRC Press), Boca Raton Fl, 1992.

Fingl E, Woodbury DM, General Principles, pg 1-59 in GoodmanLS, Gilman A, THE PHARMACOLOGICAL BASIS OF THERAPEUTICS, 5th Ed, Macmillan Publ, NY, 1975

TOTAL LOAD

Black CM, Welsh KI, Occupationally and Environmentally Induced Scleroderma-Like Illness: Etiology, Pathogenesis, Diagnosis, and Treatment. INTERNAL MEDICINE 9:6 135-154, June 1988.

The title of this paper sums it up. Because here we have a disease like scleroderma that is a medical enigma: no known cause, no known cure and no effective treatment without serious side effects. Yet when one applies the principles of environmental medicine, this all changes. It opens up a whole new world of health possibilities.

The total body burden of stressors must be dealt with in order to sufficiently unload the body and allow it to heal. But when you deal with drug-oriented medicine and only one symptom or organ at a time (because of our fabricated system of medical specialization), this concept is new to many.

But it is not so strange. If someone has a cycle accident and suffers a nasty gash full of road dirt, we don't just suture it. Instead, we lower the total load as much as possible to allow optimal healing. We anesthetize the area, scrub it up, x-ray for fractures, boost tetanus, splint it or put the injured part or patient to rest, and may even prescribe an antibiotic. We do whatever it takes to assure optimal healing.

Likewise, when you are dealing with multiple symptoms and trying to identify cause, a more exacting history is needed (see History section). Then specialized allergen testing, usually with the fine-tuned titration method, which is more suited to the potentially dangerously sensitive individual and is far safer (see SDET references).

Since food sensitivity can mimic nearly any symptom as well, various diets will be evaluated. Food testing and injections are used only if necessary. Nutrient deficiencies can be judiciously sought since they too, can mimic any symptom. In addition, they are so prevalent and underly all pathology.

Next, depending on symptoms and outcome from these, if wellness is still elusive and there are bowel complaints, a check for the hyperpermeable gut and intestinal dysbiosis might be in order. For either of these can be the underlying cause for many systemic as well as organ-specific symptoms from Crohn's disease or to rheumatoid arthritis to elusive fatigue or multiple escalating allergies.

Hormone deficiencies, and general standard medical conditions may need to be ruled out, as well.

And last but not least, a myriad of chemical sensitivities and toxicities can mimic any symptom. And one of the most surreptitious yet ubiquitous of these are pesticides. By identifying and avoiding these, or taking measures to improve the detoxication of xenobiotics, one can reduce symptoms.

Likewise, undetected pesticide exposures, for example, can "rapidly deplete cellular mechanisms", and "enzyme inductions can increase the overall rate of biotransformation of a chemical, which can in turn lead to an excess production of reactive intermediates". "And these doses need not be large, for detoxication pathways are compromised and non-toxic doses of a xenobiotic (foreign chemical) can now result in cellular injury".

In other words if possible chemical culprits are not sought, a variety of metabolic defects can result with escalation of further "undiagnosable" and "untreatable" symptoms. For if the total load of environmental stressors and biochemical defects is not addressed, the patient invariably develops additional diagnostic problems as more damage accumulates in the system. Timely diagnosis and treatment can forestall an irreversible or fatal worsening.

Sipes G, Gandolfi AJ, Biotransformation of Toxicants, in Klaasen CD, Amdur MD, Doul J, CASARETT & DOULL'S TOXICOLOGY, 3rd ed, Macmillan Publ, NY 1986.

Likewise, many conditions, like scleroderma, for example, are supposed to have no known cause or cure. But chemical exposures have been the trigger (reference at beginning of this section). The point is that regardless of how enigmatic a particular condition has always been, once you start applying the rules of environmental medicine, many "impossible" conditions heal.

Addressing the total load is one of the principles that is difficult for some non-environmentally trained physicians, who are accustomed to prescribing one or two drugs for a symptom or disease and calling it quits. Focus and knowledge cannot be restricted to one target organ, for all complaints of the patient, mental and physical, need to be addressed in order to find cause.

Classic examples abound in the failure to address the total load and how it sentences the patient to a lifetime of drugs that actually accelerate the underlying pathology: (1) the rheumatologist who does not address the gastrointestinal tract to look for hidden food allergies, intestinal hyperpermeability or intestinal dysbiosis, or (2) the cardiologist who does not address nutrient deficiencies and chemical sensitivities.

110

These types of organ-centered drug-oriented physicians who do not address the total load are actually accelerating their patients' illnesses. For example, if the patients' arthritis is caused by a food allergy which in turn was promoted because of a leaky gut syndrome, which was triggered by intestinal dysbiosis, then the last thing the patient needs is an NSAID. But NSAIDs (non-steroidal anti-inflamatory drugs) are the first line of treatment by these physicians. Yet the literature is replete with references of how NSAids cause the leaky gut, not to mention fatal haemorrhage. So the mechanism that causes the symptoms is being perpetuated by the very drug chosen to cover or mask the symptom.

Likewise look at the simple example of an individual who has an intracellular deficiency of magnesium and manganese, who may present to the cardiologist with arrhythmia. But when a calcium channel blocker is prescribed this indicates that the physician has overlooked the fact that magnesium is nature's calcium channel blocker. And its deficiency cannot be found without a proper loading test, and it will not correct if there is a concomitant manganese deficiency. And if uncorrected (which using the current serum magnesium test and prescribing drugs fosters) can progress to sudden cardiac arrest. (References for all these scenarios are in the preceding sections.)

In essence, by resorting to drugs to mask or control symptoms, we often cause the sick to get sicker, quicker.

The key Is Finding the Cause, Not the Label

With all the knowledge that the study of environmental medicine has provided, it has become clear that the key to wellness is finding the cause of symptoms, not just finding a label for a constellation of symptoms that can then only be drugged.

Regardless of which target organ is looked at, clinicians from all aspects of medicine are stumbling into environmental medicine by identifying the causes of conditions that prior were enigmas with no known cause of treatment:

Abuelo JG, Renal failure caused by chemicals, foods, plants, animal venoms, and misuse of drugs. An overview, ARCH INTERN MED, 50: 505-510, 1990.

Acute pancreatitis following cutaneous exposure to an organophosphate insecticide, INTERN MED WORLD REP, P 10, Mar 1-14, 1989 (Marsh et al, AMER J GASTROENT 83: 1158-1160, 1988).

Straus SE, Dale JK, Wright R, Metcalfe DD, Allergy and the chronic fatigue syndrome, J ALLERGY CLIN IMMUNOL 1988: 81: 791-5

NOTES ON INDIVIDUAL DISEASES

You can begin to see that looking for the environmental trigger and the biochemical defect applies to nearly everything, but there are certain common formulas that we use for specific diseases. For example, in working up simple perennial allergic rhinitis, often we will just test to the common pollens, dusts and molds that are in the ambient area after having taken a history from the patient.

The same goes for reversible obstructive airway disease or asthma, although those people often have to do the diagnostic diet as well, because hidden food sensitivities are so commonly a part of this symptom. Likewise, asthmatics need to do, bare minimum, a magnesium loading test, as magnesium deficiency has been found to be one of the contributory factors to bronchospasm.

Likewise, people with irritable bowel syndrome need diets and usually nutrient tests because of accelerated loss of nutrients from diarrhea and an inflamed bowel. The toxic encephalopathy or brain fog obviously requires bare minimum looking at some nutrient levels that are common in the detoxification pathway, since the inability to properly detoxify chemicals comes about when nutrients such as intracellular zinc, molybdenum, manganese, and copper are deficient in the xenobiotic detoxification pathway (remember the chemistry of "brain fog" in the trichloroethylene section).

Chronic fatigue entails looking at multiple nutrients, but again we try to be judicious and pick the most likely ones. And so on it goes - headache, migraine, muscle spasms, chemical sensitivities, atopic dermatitis, hypertension, depression, hypercholesterolemia or hyperlipidemia, arthritis, osteoporosis, diabetes, hypoglycemia, epilepsy, cancer, chronic low back pain, cardiac arrhythmia, chronic cystitis, chronic prostatitis, or what have you. We really do not care what the diagnostic label is so much as finding what is **causing** the symptoms. For most all symptoms have multiple environmental triggers and biochemical defects that can usually be identified and corrected.

REASONS INSURANCE COMPANIES
USE TO REJECT CLAIMS

What necessitated this monograph is akin to what two episodes of the television documentary "60 Minutes" devoted itself to: the unethical and illegal practices of some insurance companies. It has been necessitated by such groups as VOICE (Victims of Insurance Company Exploitation). The intent is to set the record straight, educate, and help innocent people who are being illegally discriminated against, and save them the cost and time of class action suits, small claims courts, contacting their state attorney general and insurance regulation board, the media, etc. For it is a belief that given the opportunity to glimpse at a smattering of the overwhelming evidence, rationale and explanation, most insurance companies are humane and ethical.

Service Not Reasonable and Customary

The first reason often listed to justify denying payment for medical care is that work-ups are not **"reasonable and customary"**. But according to the 6/13/90 **Journal of the American Medical Association,** 90% of physicians fail to even look for a magnesium deficiency in patients so sick as to be hospitalized and 54% of these patients were deficient and many of them died of the undiagnosed deficiency. Thus it is customary for doctors to be dangerously poor in nutritional biochemistry. But it is not excusable nor a rational reason to reject those patients whose physicians are knowledgeable.

Although the cited JOURNAL OF THE AMERICAN MEDICAL ASSOCIATION study shows that you can die from medical practice that is "reasonable and customary", this study does not stand alone. There are numerous studies that prove that the customary practice of medicine is dan-

115

gerously below par. For example in the AMERICAN JOUR-
NAL OF CARDIOLOGY they showed that of 143 patients
admitted to a regional coronary care unit, 40% were low in
magnesium. And the pitiful part was they used the worst,
least sensitive assay, a **serum** magnesium, to make this
determination! That means that more than 40% were low.

Seelig CB, Montano CE, Ranney JE, physician recognition
of magnesium status in patients with coronary artery disease admitted to a regional medical center. AMER J
CARDIOL 72: 226-227, July 15, 1993.

Likewise the U.S. Department of Health and Human Services published a report that only 2% of charts include
information regarding toxic exposures, duration of present
employment and former occupation. As for reasonable-
ness, this same government agency makes it explicitly clear
that the inclusion of an environmental history is the gold
standard of good medicine; and you don't collect this
information just to collect data. An environmental history
is a necessary part of the diagnosis and subsequent treatment. Again, being "customary"(to omit environmental
considerations) does not excuse it and in no way should
exempt the patient from insurance coverage.

Furthermore, many patients have disease and symptoms
that resist diagnosis. They have consulted over a dozen
certified specialists and have had all that is "reasonable and
customary" done. But it did not help them. Do their con-
tracts state that if they have a difficult case, that it exempts
their company from coverage? The more difficult the medical problem, the more likely that there is an environmental
medicine solution. If you have a medical problem that is not
customary, then mde than likely neither will the treatment
or solution be customary. Likewise, the more physians a
person has to consult, with no answers, the more likely that

116

the final solution will not be customary. This is not a reason to penalize or discriminate against the patient who has a difficult problem.

Unproven and Experimental

The next term that is commonly used to deny payments is calling the technique **"unproven and experimental"**. They use this to reject SDET (serial dilution end-point titration, or simply titrated extracts). Yet there are no studies to disprove SDET. And it has been used for over half of a century, and is currently used by over 2000 physicians. And there are no reports of adverse reactions. Bt there is a plethora of articles substantiating its benefits and scientific merits. And the many cited articles documenting death as the outcome when non-titrated antigens are used.

And when this phrase is used to reject food or chemical testing via (P-N) provocation-neutralization, recall that this stems from the American Academy of Allergy and Immunology whose **only** rebuttal is an outrageously flawed study. They actually mistakenly used the dose that causes or provokes symptoms in place of the dose that turns them off or treats them.

To use this phrase in regard to SDET or P-N serves only to alert one to the fact that the medical advisors are ignorant of the scores of references and the fact that there have been no serious adverse reactions as there have been with the less than individualized "canned" approach that conventional allergy uses to tests patients. And remember that the **Journal of the American Medical Association** stated that serial dilution titration is indeed a very useful and scientific modality. In fact all of quantitative science is based on titration, as it is the only way to be accurate. And what better place to be accurate than when injecting potentially

117

lethal substances into highly allergic and sensitive people.

And if class action patients wanted to hire an attorney to subpoena claims from insurance companies, they would find that many unproven technologies are covered by insurance companies. Many prescription drugs, for example, chemotherapy, are not only experimental, but are known for failure, yet they are covered. In fact, statistics show that the chances of long-term and meaningful survival on the majority of these protocols is extremely slim, yet they are covered. Furthermore, for the vast majority of drugs in the PDR (PHYSICIANS DESK REFERENCE) the "mechanism of action is unknown". Now **that** is experimental.

In addition, as another United States government service tells us, insurance companies do underwrite expensive medical treatments that are totally experimental like bone marrow transplants for breast cancers which cost well in excess of $100,000. Not only is this experimental, but the patient has a 1 in 3 chance of dying of the procedure itself. Is that good odds for that kind of money?

Let's look at a quote from Cancer Fax from the National Cancer Institute, p.1

"In 1991, the National Cancer Institute began sponsoring randomized clinical trials of high-dose chemotherapy with autologous bone marrow transplant." "In a break with insurance industry practice, the Blue Cross and Blue Shield Association announced an innovative demonstration project to help support clinical care costs of these trials. The clinical trials will enroll approximately 1,500 women."

Cancer Fax 1-301-402-5874

And it is ironic that there are cases of cancer of the breast that have had bone marrow transplants and chemotherapy and all of these have been failures. These patients have been given up on by physicians and told that they had as little as two weeks to live. They then went on diets that turned around their conditions and they cleared their cancers. But no one wants to investigate this or even pay for their inexpensive supplements. This is in spite of published papers proving that the diets have healed cancers when all else that high tech medicine can offer has failed and that inexpensive nutrients more than halved the cancer recurrence rates.

(JACN, Carter, et al, 12:3, 1993 and J UROL, Lamm D, et al, Jan 1994).

Or take the coverage of AZT for HIV when double-blind studies in 3 countries showed "there was no statistically significant or clinically important benefit in terms of disease progression or survival from the immediate use of zidovudine":

Concorde Coordinating Committee: Concorde: MRC/ANRS randomized double-blind controlled trial of immediate and deferred zidovudine in symptom-free HIV infection. LANCET 1994; 343:871

Likewise, "the use of the methacholine inhalational challenge (MCH) has become widely accepted as a clinical tool to evaluate patients who are first seen with respiratory symptoms suggestive of asthma". However, "cough persisted in almost 50% of both methacholine - positive and methacholine - negative groups". Furthermore, "symptoms of chest tightness, wheezing, and shortness of breath were present during follow-up in a surprising number of subjects with negative MCH results, and within the methacholine - positive group, there was poor correlation among the degree of airway responsiveness, clinical symptoms, and ongoing treatment". In other words, the test is worthless, but nevertheless widely performed and covered, especially in many medical centers.

Muller BA, Leich CA, Prognostic Value of Methacholine Challenge in Patients with Respiratory Symptoms. J ALLERGY CLIN IMMUNOL 1994; 94:77-87.

A final note on this reason for rejection: There are many physicians whose SDET is covered by insurance companies, while the same technique is not covered when performed by other physicians. There appears to be an arbitrary discrimination against those not covered, as they tend to all be members of a specific medical organization. In other words there is strong evidence that this decision is one based on medical politics, not scientific facts.

The bottom line is there are wide arbitrary and capricious discrepancies and inconsistencies in what is called experimental and what is covered. And there is gross lack of familiarity with the science on which these decisions are supposedly based.

Not Commonly Done

Another reason used for rejection by insurance companies is that the techniques are **not commonly done** by the vast number of physicians. But this is certainly understandable because the vast number of physicians are drug oriented and do not utilize sophisticated biochemistry. As government studies show, 98% of physicians do not do an adequate environmental history! So does this mean that patients lucky or smart enough or sick enough to go to the 2% who do should be penalized?

First of all who wants to be relegated to the lowest level of competency in your neighborhood anyway? If the majority of physicians are out playing golf, why must patients be penalized for consulting someone who has extraordinary knowledge who is able help them clear conditions in a drug-free manner?

Secondly, these patients have already fallen through the cracks and defied diagnosis. So they are all difficult to diagnose patients. Just because a majority of physicians cannot diagnose them, does not mean that they should be denied coverage while others with more easily recognizable labels have their treatments paid for. Is the insurance company saying it only covers simple straight-forward conditions that every doctor can diagnose and that respond to drugs? In fact it does not matter if the ddrug does not have a good cure rate (chemotherapy). Results seem to be inconsequential. This is mindless cookbook or computerized medicine that eventually leads to further and faster breakdown of the body, by not finding and fixing the underlying defect. A headache is not an aspirin deficiency, and there are no studies to prove this. Yet it is the basis of medical care that is covered by some companies.

I do not recall an insurance contract that ever stated that a patient would be denied payment if ten out of ten physicians did not know what to do for him. Nor have I seen a statement that he would be denied coverage if his condition necessitated consulting a particularly innovative or specialized physician, or that he would be denied coverage if only one out of 10 physicians could make him well. Yet that is what this reason for rejection implies.

The Senate has recently investigated Blue Cross & Blue Shield Insurance. "Investigators testified at a Senate subcommittee hearing" after a 2 year probe, that BC/BS has

121

spent millions of dollars each year in "excessive salaries, conferences, and meeting expenses as well as gifts such as neon shoelaces and balloons".

Last year the President, Bernard Trenowski, had a salary of $866,000, while in 1992 the West Virginia Plan was declared insolvent. Exposed were "extravagant spending on travel by executives, a series of mismanaged subsidiaries", and "non-standard accounting methods to show a healthy plan to the public".

Staff & Wire Reports: Senate Report Blasts Blue Cross, High Salaries, Expenses Detailed. 13c, 21c THE SUN, Baltimore MD, Sat., Aug 6, 1994

As well, by denying coverage for an environmental medicine approach to diagnosis and treatment, insurance companies do not even exhibit good common sense. For example, studies in the JOURNAL OF THE AMERICAN COLLEGE OF NUTRITION (Carter, et al 12:3, 209, 1993) show that if you do everything medicine has to offer for cancer of the prostate (surgery, chemotherapy, radiation, hormones), the median survival is 6 years. However, if you save $100,000 and merely do the macrobiotic diet, median survival is not 6 years, but 19 years. There is no contest. But BC/BS pays for the former and not for the latter.

Likewise, the study in THE LANCET showed 59 patients whose mean age was 82, all of whom were in the hospital for a hip fracture. They all had the same treatment except half of them received a multiple vitamin/mineral. That group had a median hospital stay of 22 days, while the non-vitamin/mineral group had a median hospital stay of 44 days. What a phenomenal medical savings. With hospital rooms averaging in excess of $800 a day, and thousands of hip fracture patients a year, this is financial management at

122

its worst.

In addition to double the hospital stay, the patients in this study who did not have supplements had twice the number of deaths and twice the complications. But prescription drugs are usually covered while physician-prescribed nutrients are not covered, even with documented deficiencies. And it takes a great deal more medical decision making, biochemical knowledge, training, and expertise to write a prescription to correct and balance biochemcial deficiencies than it does to copy one drug and its dose from the PDR.

Likewise, a study in the JOURNAL OF UROLOGY (Lamm D, Jan. 1994) showed that if you do everything medicine has to offer for a certain type of bladder cancer, for example, that in 2 years it all comes back in 80% of the victims. But when they gave 4 simple vitamins, the recurrence rate dropped in half to 40%. But that is not covered.

Furthermore, many insurance companies sponsor prescription drug plans where they force people to get 3 months' of a prescription even when they are only going to use 2 weeks of it. For example, Claritin is a newer antihistamine and costs around $186.00 per bottle of 100. But if a person has a plan, he is urged to get 3 months worth even though he only needs it 2-3 weeks during the flowering of a particular tree.

Then the same insurance company will often deny coverage for correction of documented vitamin and mineral deficiencies in people who have exhausted all that medicine has to offer. This is even after correction of the deficiencies has solved their health problems, enabled them to get off costly ineffective medications, and get back to work.

Clearly some factions of the insurance business are not

123

interested in what is scientifically valid, nor what is common sense or logical. They appear to be dedicated to high-tech costly surgery and drugs. Investigative reporters, Senate Investigational Subcommittees and TV documentaries have substantiated this and more. This is what has necessitated a monograph such as this, so that victims of unjust insurance discrimination will be armed with evidence in order to receive what they have worked and paid for.

PREVENTATIVE MEDICINE NOT COVERED

Sometimes a reason for rejection is that the service is considered part of preventative medicine, and preventative medicine is not covered. But all of medicine is preventive.

Coronary bypass surgery is to prevent or postpone death. An appendectomy is done to prevent rupture and peritonitis. Reduction of an open or compound fracture is done to prevent infection and faulty union. High blood pressure medicine and cholesterol-lowering medicines are an attempt to prevent or delay the onset of further symptoms of arteriosclerosis.

But the underlying defect in all pathologies, from cancer, arteriosclerosis, arthritis, stroke, heart attacks, cataracts and even aging is oxidation, better known as free radical-induced lipid peroxidation. And nutrient prescriptions can ameliorate this.

Halliwell B, Gutteridge JMC, FREE RADICALS IN BIOLOGY AND MEDICINE, Clarendon, Oxford, 1985

Cerutti PA, Prooxidant states and tumor promotion, SCIENCE, 227: 375-381, 1985

Cross CE, Halliwell Borish ET, Pryor WA, Ames BN, Saul RL, McCord JM, Harmon D, Oxygen radicals and human diseases, ANN INTERN MED, 107: 526-545, 1987.

Even every lay person has heard of the 1993 NEW ENGLAND JOURNAL OF MEDICINE study (Stampfer, et al, 328: 1444-1449, 1993) on 85,000 people showing that a paltry 100 I.U. of vitamin E a day cuts the cardiovascular risk in half. And this is the number one cause of death and disease in the U.S. But numerous other scientific works show temendously more the importance of treating the underlying biochemcial defect rather than masking the symptom with drugs.

For example, the JOURNAL OF THE AMERICAN MEDICAL ASSOCIATION tells is that "In national surveys, a substantial proportion of the U.S. population consumes levels of several vitamins that are well below the recommended intakes, and recent evidence strongly indicated that such low intakes are associated with serious health consequences." This was from the Harvard Medical School of Public Health.

Stampfer MJ, Willett WC, Homocysteine and marginal vitamin deficiency, The importance of adequate vitamin intake, J AMER MED ASSOC, 270:22, 2726-2727, Dec 8, 1993.

These Harvard public health medical specialists go on to show how a vast number of people, for example are low in folic acid and that this undetected, uncorrected deficiency can go on to contribute to the number one health problem, arteriosclerosis. And many journals show how it prevents neural tube defects, a problem that sentences the parents of these babies to medical costs in the hundreds of thousands.

Likewise, if you look at vitamin C, it has an important function in lowering cholesterol and changing it into bile acids. Then it is excreted through the liver and bile ducts into the gut. When this happens, it is attached to harmful daily chemicals and drags them out of the body as well. So when you treat high cholesterol, not with drugs but from its biochemical origins, you are at the same time doing other beneficial things for the body, like fascilitating xenobiotic (foreign chemical) detoxification.

Ginter E, Cholesterol: Vitamin C controls its transformation to bile acids, SCIENCE, 179: 4074, 702-704, Feb 16, 1973.

And vitamin C, as an example of one tiny function of only one of over 40 essential nutrients, is the strongest aqueous phase (outside of the cell) anti-oxidant in the body. Translation: This brings us full cycle back to one of its main functions, that of negating or neutralizing the very chemistry that underlies all diseases. In essence, it is the epitomy of biochemical ignorance to resort to drug therapy before trying to identify and correct the underlying biochemical/nutritional defects.

Frei B, England L, Ames BN, Ascorbate is an outstanding antioxidant in human blood plasma, PROC NATL ACAD SCI, 86: 6377-6381, 1989.

PHONE CONSULTATIONS

When patients travel well over 100 miles to see a physician, there are obvious advantages to being able to to follow up with phone conversations. Phone consultations save patients the time and money of taking a day off from work, getting baby-sitters and the time and money spent in traveling and waiting in a doctor's office. As well, some patients have to travel so far to a specialized physician, that they need to stay over night. This further adds to expense of the visit.

In the specialty of environmental medicine, there is a major empowerment of the patient. And the only way this empowerment can be effective is if there is a tremendous amount of patient education. Environmental controls, diet counseling, and how to take nutrient prescriptions for a deficiency are all things that patients need instruction for. These can be done on the telephone just as well as in the office since there is no physical examination needed.

For example, when nutrient levels have been drawn and deficiencies have been identified, it is necessary to have a patient-physician consultation to go over the deficiencies, explain how they occcured, how they are going to be corrected, how to take the individualized biochemical plan that has been created for that patient, and what caveats to watch for. This can be done just as well on the telephone as in the office. And the beauty of it is people do not need to spend the time and the money away from work, plus travelling (and overnight lodging) to the physician's office.

Many patients with difficult conditions have had to travel hundreds of miles to find a specialist in environmental medicine and popping back to the office every few months would be impractical. But scheduled phone visits, treated just the same as an office visit, are highly effective. A last benefit of the phone consultation in place of the office visit is that some chemically sensitive people are too ill to be exposed to auto exhaust and commercial travel (and lodging). They have spent a great deal of money, often, in creating a home environment in which to heal, and it can be counterproductive for them to leave it prematurely.

PRESCRIPTIONS FOR NON-PRESCRIPTION ITEMS

There are many items that do not require prescriptions, but which are prescribed by physicians. Iron deficiency, folic acid deficiency are examples. Other things include various appliances, air cleaners, canes, walkers, wheel chairs, orthotics or braces, etc.

In the case of nutrient deficiencies, for example, there are usually documented biochemical defects, like a magnesium deficiency. These deficiencies are crucial to correct with knowledge that only a physician would possess. They constitute the very "nuts and bolts" of how the body functions in health. It is inconceivable that an insurance company would not pay for a physician-prescribed correction of a deficiency, that has such far ranging effects on health if left uncorrected. It takes far more biochemical knowledge and medical decision making by the physician to correct these deficiencies than it does to prescribe a medication from the PDR.

Medications merely mask the symptoms and are not tailored to the biochemistry of the individual person, as a nutrient prescription after assaying the key nutrients is.

Let's look at one example, L-carnitine, a simple, harmless, non-prescription body constituent. Yet in spite of numerous papers detailing its medical benefits, most physicians have never heard of it. Yet it can enable a patient to reduce his need for heart drugs like digitalis and diuretics (which do have harmful side effects that can include death). It increases the energy source of the heart (promotes the transfer of acetyl CoA to the mitochondria of heart muscle cells). It lowers cholesterol (by restoring fatty acid metabolism). It can improve the heart rate, congestive heart failure, edema, shortness of breath and more.

So here we have, as an example of one non-prescription necessary body constituent, something that is

* inexpensive,
* has no side effects,
* is safer than the drugs it displaces,
* can improve the cardiac status beyond what is possible with drugs,
* costs less, and
* can save lives, above and beyond what can be done with drugs.

But it is considered not necessary to be covered because it is

* non-prescription
* most doctors do not use it (not usual and customary), and
* most doctors have been heard of it

It appears that an investigation into why an insurance company would want to perpetuate disease and discriminate in favor of the pharmaceutical industry would be in order in these cases. For there is no logical or ethical explanation.

Ghidini O, Azzurro M, Vita G, Sartori G, Evaluation of the therapeutic efficacy of L-canitine in congestive heart failure, INTERN J CLIN PHARMACOL, THER & TOXICOL, 26:4, 217-220, 1988

THE NEED FOR SPECIAL HOUSING WHILE TESTING

Some patients are so ill with chemical sensitivity, that they can not stay in commercial buildings with carpeting, air fresheners, strong cleansers, pesticides, smokers, etc. These people need special environmentally controlled housing with air cleaners, wood floors, cotton bedding and other amenities. This special housing is available at some clinics for people too ill to tolerate commercial lodgings.

SUMMARY

It should be abundantly clear from this very abbreviated short monograph for patients, attorneys, small claims courts, attorney generals, insurance investigators and many more, that there is voluminous evidence to support looking for the cause of conditions and symptoms, rather than prescribing a lifetime of drugs to merely mask the symptoms. There is a vast amount of data that has not been presented. It should be clear that this approach is the logical, medically correct, and the ethical thing to do, as it results in overall healthier people and at a lower cost. And it fosters the development of adults who become in part responsible for their health. Remember, the United States Department of Health and Human Services Public Health Service says, "Unless an exposure history is pursued by the physician, the etiologic diagnosis may be missed, treatment may be inappropriate and exposure may continue".

ADDENDUM

As more problems arise with insurances and more evidence is needed, there will be updates for this monograph available through Sand Key Publications, Box 40101, Sarasota, FL 34242. Please send your name and address if you would like to be put on the mailing list.

130